om

Agnes E. Rupley, DVM

CONSULTING EDITOR

VETERINARY CLINICS

OF NORTH AMERICA

Exotic Animal Practice

Gastroenterology

GUEST EDITOR
Tracey K. Ritzman, DVM, Dipl. ABVP–Avian

May 2005 • Volume 8 • Number 2

SAUNDERS

An Imprint of Elsevier, Inc.
PHILADELPHIA   LONDON   TORONTO   MONTREAL   SYDNEY   TOKYO

W.B. SAUNDERS COMPANY
A Division of Elsevier Inc.

The Curtis Center • Independence Square West • Philadelphia, Pennsylvania 19106

http://www.vetexotic.theclinics.com

THE VETERINARY CLINICS OF NORTH AMERICA: Volume 8, Number 2
EXOTIC ANIMAL PRACTICE   ISSN 1094-9194
May 2005   ISBN 1-4160-2834-X
Editor: John Vassallo

The ideas and opinions expressed in *The Veterinary Clinics of North America: Exotic Animal Practice* do not necessarily reflect those of the Publisher. The Publisher does not assume any responsibility for any injury and/or damage to persons or property arising out of or related to any use of the material contained in this periodical. The reader is advised to check the appropriate medical literature and the product information currently provided by the manufacturer of each drug to be administered to verify the dosage, the method and duration of administration, or contraindications. It is the responsibility of the treating physician or other health care professional, relying on independent experience and knowledge of the patient, to determine drug dosages and the best treatment for the patient. Mention of any product in this issue should not be construed as endorsement by the contributors, editors, or the Publisher of the product or manufacturers' claims.

The Veterinary Clinics of North America: Exotic Animal Practice (ISSN 1094-9194) is published in January, May, and September by W.B. Saunders Company; Corporate and editorial offices: The Curtis Center, Independence Square West, Philadelphia, PA 19106-3399. Accounting and circulation offices: 6277 Sea Harbor Drive, Orlando, FL 32887-4800. Subscription prices are $130.00 per year for US individuals, $215.00 per year for US institutions, $65.00 per year for US students and residents, $156.00 per year for Canadian individuals, $250.00 per year for Canadian institutions, $165.00 per year for international individuals, $250.00 per year for international institutions and $83.00 per year for Canadian and foreign students/residents. To receive student/resident rate, orders must be accompanied by name of affiliated institution, date of term, and the *signature* of program/residency coordinator on institution letterhead. Orders will be billed at individual rate until proof of status is received. Foreign air speed delivery is included in all *Clinics* subscription prices. All prices are subject to change without notice.

POSTMASTER: Send address changes to *The Veterinary Clinics of North America: Exotic Animal Practice*; W.B. Saunders Company, Periodicals Fulfillment, Orlando, FL 32887-4800. **Customer Service: 1-800-654-2452 (US). From outside of the US, call 1-407-345-1000.**

The Veterinary Clinics of North America: Exotic Animal Practice is covered in *Index Medicus*.

Printed in the United States of America.

GOAL STATEMENT

The goal of the *Veterinary Clinics of North America: Exotic Animal Practice* is to keep practicing veterinarians up to date with current clinical practice in exotic animal medicine by providing timely articles reviewing the state of the art in exotic animal care.

ACCREDITATION

The *Veterinary Clinics of North America: Exotic Animal Practice* will be offering continuing education credits, to be awarded by a school of veterinary medicine, contract pending.

The aforementioned school of veterinary medicine is a designated a provider of continuing veterinary education. Veterinarians participating in this learning activity may earn up to 6 credits per issue or a maximum of 18 credits per year. Credits awarded may not apply toward license renewal in all states. It is the responsibility of each participant to verify the requirements of their state licensing board.

Credit can be earned by reading the text material, taking the examination online at *http://www. theclinics.com/home/cme*, and completing the program evaluation. Each test question must be answered correctly; you will have the opportunity to retake any questions answered incorrectly. Following successful completion of the test and the program evaluation, you may print your certificate.

TO ENROLL

To enroll in the *Veterinary Clinics of North America: Exotic Animal Practice* Continuing Education program, call customer service at 1-800-654-2452 or sign up online at *http://www.theclinics.com/home/ cme*. The CME program is available to subscribers for an additional annual fee of $49.95.

CONSULTING EDITOR

AGNES E. RUPLEY, DVM, Diplomate, American Board of Veterinary
Practitioners-Avian Practice; and Director and Chief Veterinarian,
All Pets Medical & Laser Surgical Center, College Station, Texas

GUEST EDITOR

TRACEY K. RITZMAN, DVM, Diplomate, American Board of Veterinary
Practitioners-Avian Practice; Staff Veterinarian, Angell Animal Medical Center, Boston,
Massachusetts

CONTRIBUTORS

JO CLANCY, Department of Small Animal Clinical Sciences, College of Veterinary
Medicine, The University of Tennessee, Knoxville, Tennessee

LEIGH ANN CLAYTON, DVM, Associate Veterinarian, National Aquarium in
Baltimore, Baltimore, Maryland

ORLANDO DIAZ-FIGUEROA, DVM, Resident, Zoological Medicine, Department
of Veterinary Clinical Sciences, Louisiana State University School of Veterinary
Medicine, Baton Rouge, Louisiana

CHRIS GRIFFIN, DVM, Diplomate, American Board of Veterinary Practitioners-
Avian Practice; Griffin Avian and Exotic Veterinary Hospital, Kannapolis, North
Carolina

JOSEPH W. GRIFFIN, JR, MD, Diplomate, American Board of Internal Medicine-
Gastroenterology; Augusta Gastroenterology Associates, Augusta, Georgia

TARAH L. HADLEY, DVM, Resident, Department of Small Animal Clinical Sciences,
College of Veterinary Medicine, The University of Tennessee, Knoxville, Tennessee

CATHY A. JOHNSON-DELANEY, DVM, Diplomate, American Board of Veterinary
Practitioners-Avian Practice; Avian and Exotics Advanced Diagnostic Consulting,
Edmonds; Exotic Pet Bird Clinic, Kirkland; Pet and Exotic Clinic of Seattle, Seattle,
Washington

ERIC KLAPHAKE, DVM, Resident, Department of Small Animal Clinical Sciences,
College of Veterinary Medicine, The University of Tennessee, Knoxville, Tennessee

ANGELA M. LENNOX, DVM, Diplomate, American Board of Veterinary Practitioners-Avian Practice; Avian and Exotic Animal Clinic of Indianapolis, Indianapolis, Indiana

MARK A. MITCHELL, DVM, MS, PhD, Assistant Professor, Zoological Medicine, Department of Veterinary Clinical Sciences, Louisiana State University School of Veterinary Medicine, Baton Rouge, Louisiana

DAVID PHALEN, DVM, PhD, Diplomate, American Board of Veterinary Practitioners-Avian Practice; Associate Professor, Schubot Exotic Bird Health Center and Department of Large Animal Clinical Sciences, College of Veterinary Medicine, Texas A&M University, College Station, Texas

BRIGITTE REUSCH, BVetMed (HONS), MRCVS, RWF Rabbit and Zoo Animal Resident, Division of Companion Animals, Department of Clinical Veterinary Science, Small Animal Hospital, University of Bristol, Langford, Bristol, United Kingdom

E. SCOTT WEBER, MSc (Aquatic Veterinary Science), VMD, Head Veterinarian and Research Scientist, Animal Health Department, Husbandry Division, New England Aquarium, Boston, Massachusetts

CONTENTS

Preface   xi
Tracey K. Ritzman

**A Glimpse of the Human Field of Gastroenterology
and Applications for Veterinary Medicine**   183
Chris Griffin and Joseph W. Griffin, Jr

> The future of veterinary gastroenterology may be greatly enhanced
> by the technologic, therapeutic, and diagnostic advancements cur-
> rently available to physicians. Capsule endoscopy, endoscopic ul-
> trasound, proton pump inhibitors, computed tomography, and
> other cutting edge techniques and therapies may become a larger
> part of veterinary medicine, and will undoubtedly lead to more ac-
> curate diagnosis and treatment of gastrointestinal disease in exotic
> pet patients.

**The Ferret Gastrointestinal Tract and *Helicobacter mustelae*
Infection**   197
Cathy A. Johnson-Delaney

> The gastrointestinal tract of the domestic ferret, *Mustela putorius
> furo*, has been studied extensively as a model for several human
> gastrointestinal tract diseases, including spontaneous gastric and
> duodenal ulcers, gastroesophageal reflux, gastric carcinoma and
> lymphoma, the lack of acid mucosubstances similar to humans,
> and *Helicobacter mustelae* infection. To discuss the implications of
> the role of *Helicobacter* in disease, we must first review the unique
> anatomy and physiology of the ferret digestive system.

Gastrointestinal Diseases of the Ferret   213
Angela M. Lennox

> Gastrointestinal disease is common in pet ferrets. Unique ferret
> anatomy and physiology predisposes ferrets to primary gastroin-
> testinal disease as well as gastrointestinal symptoms secondary

to stress or general debilitation. Identification of etiology can be difficult, and requires a thorough diagnostic approach, as many gastrointestinal disease conditions produce similar symptoms. A combination of traditional diagnostic modalities, plus newer novel diagnostic tests, can aid in both diagnosis and optimal therapeutic management of ferrets with gastrointestinal disease.

Amphibian Gastroenterology 227
Leigh Ann Clayton

This article begins with a review of gastrointestinal anatomy of larval and adult anurans (frogs, toads) and urodeles (salamanders, newts, sirens). A brief discussion of clinical signs and diagnostic tools is included. Common disease and treatment options also are discussed.

Gastroenterology for the Piscine Patient 247
E. Scott Weber

Fish are the largest group of vertebrates, and with estimates of species at 25,000, piscine patients pose a great veterinary challenge for private practice, on fish farms, and in a public aquarium setting. This article reviews the piscine gastrointestinal tract beginning with the mouth and food apprehension, through the stomach, intestines, pyloric cecae, and with discussion on accessory organs. Basic anatomy of each gastrointestinal tract section with some pertinent histologic considerations and some general physiologic considerations is discussed. This article also includes diagnostic modalities frequently used to investigate gastrointestinal disease in fish, which include ultrasound, radiography, contrast radiography, fecal testing, cloacal lavage, microbiology, endoscopy, and surgery.

Clinical Reptile Gastroenterology 277
Mark A. Mitchell and Orlando Diaz-Figueroa

Gastroenterology represents an important specialty within clinical reptile medicine. Veterinarians should become familiar with the unique anatomic and physiologic differences between reptiles to improve their management of these cases. In addition, veterinarians should use available diagnostic tests to confirm the presence of gastrointestinal disease. With the current advancements in reptile medicine, there is no reason these cases cannot be pursued to their fullest.

Diagnosis and Management of *Macrorhabdus ornithogaster* (Formerly Megabacteria) 299
David Phalen

Macrorhabdus ornithogaster (formerly megabacteria) is a long, thin, rigid, gram-positive yeast that grows in chains of up to four cells.

It has been identified in ostriches, chickens, and many species of wild and captive psittacine and passerine birds. Most infections with *M ornithogaster* are asymptomatic. Infection that results in disease, however, does occur in some individuals of some species, particularly canaries, finches, budgerigars, and parrotlets. Diagnosis of infection in the live bird is done by detecting the organisms in the droppings in a wet mount or stained smear. Many infected birds, however, do not shed organisms and there is material in the feces that can resemble this organism closely. Amphotericin B is the only drug that is effective for treating *M ornithogaster*.

Raptor Gastroenterology 307
Eric Klaphake and Jo Clancy

Raptors have some unique features to their gastrointestinal anatomy and physiology compared with more commonly seen birds in veterinary practices. Diseases such as trichomoniasis, lead toxicity, and herpesvirus infections need to be correctly diagnosed and treated. Management of raptor patients also presents challenges in terms of hospitalization, diagnostics, and therapeutics.

Disorders of the Psittacine Gastrointestinal Tract 329
Tarah L. Hadley

The psittacine gastrointestinal tract (GI) is a complex organ system susceptible to a variety of diseases. Disorders of the psittacine GI tract also represent some of the most challenging to diagnose and treat by the avian practitioner. The anatomy and physiology of the GI tract as it pertains to psittacine bird species will be discussed. This article will also review the most common diseases of the GI tract seen in clinical practice and the approach toward diagnosis and treatment of these diseases.

Rabbit Gastroenterology 351
Brigitte Reusch

Disorders of the oral cavity, esophagus, stomach, and intestines are important causes of disease in the rabbit. Diet-related disease and stress-related disease predominate, and can play a large role in preventive medicine. However, bacterial, viral, parasitic, idiopathic, and neoplastic diseases are also seen frequently in the domestic rabbit. Presumptive diagnosis is often created on recognition of the historic information, physical examination findings, and clinical signs. Definitive diagnosis and therapy can be challenging, although aggressive and early treatment will optimize a successful outcome.

Index 377

FORTHCOMING ISSUES

September 2005

    Practice Management
    Angela Lennox, DVM, Dipl. ABVP-Avian
    Guest Editor

January 2006

    Renal Disease
    Scott Echols, DVM, Dipl. ABVP-Avian
    Guest Editor

RECENT ISSUES

January 2005

    Virology
    Cheryl B. Greenacre, DVM, Dipl. ABVP-Avian
    Guest Editor

September 2004

    Oncology
    Jennifer E. Graham, DVM, Dipl. ABVP-Avian
    Guest Editor

May 2004

    Exotic Pet Management for the Technician
    Michelle S. Schulte, RVT, and
    Agnes E. Rupley, DVM, Dipl. ABVP-Avian
    Guest Editors

ELSEVIER
SAUNDERS

Vet Clin Exot Anim 8 (2005) xi–xii

VETERINARY
CLINICS
Exotic Animal Practice

Preface

Gastroenterology

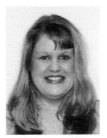

Tracey K. Ritzman, DVM, DABVP-Avian
Guest Editor

Gastroenterology is an exciting and emerging field both in human and veterinary practice. Disorders and diseases of the gastrointestinal system are an integral part of the veterinarian clinician's daily work with exotic companion animals. For the clinician working with nontraditional species, the range of presenting signs, clinical syndromes, and differential diagnoses can be quite varied and potentially overwhelming. This issue of *Veterinary Clinics of North America: Exotic Animal Practice* provides a thorough look at the gastrointestinal system and disease syndromes in birds, reptiles, small mammals, amphibians, and fish species.

The introductory article gives the reader a fascinating and provocative glimpse into the field of human gastroenterology. This article is a collaborative work by a related pair of clinicians, Drs. J. Griffin (father, an MD) and C. Griffin (son, a DVM). These authors give the reader a look at the progressive diagnostic modalities and treatment options in the field of human gastroenterology in the hope of fostering discussion and development of techniques for exotic veterinary patients.

Of all the exotic animal species, the ferret is one of the most susceptible animals to gastrointestinal derangements. This susceptibility has lead to the use of this species for human gastrointestinal research into ulcerative gastrointestinal disease, using the ferret *Helicobacter mustalea* as a model for human *Helicobacter pylori* infection and treatment. Dr. Johnson-Delaney has written a very informative article on this very topic, which includes an update on current research findings. Another article, written by Dr. Lennox, provides a comprehensive review of the myriad other gastrointestinal diseases of ferrets.

doi:10.1016/j.cvex.2005.01.006   *vetexotic.theclinics.com*

Avian patients with their unique anatomical adaptations have their own set of gastrointestinal ailments. The reader is provided with a comprehensive look at the disease syndromes of psittacines and raptors, two avian species groups frequently treated.

An update on *Macrorhabdus ornithogaster* infection and its effects on the gastrointestinal system of birds is also included.

Piscine and amphibian species are addressed as well. An enormous range of diverse species is represented in these groups of animals, and the reader will be brought up to date on the anatomy, physiology, and disease syndromes in these aquatic/amphibious patients. A section on reptiles provides an interesting look into the interesting anatomic differences this patient group possesses.

As the number of pet rabbits continues to increase, the veterinary clinician will continue to have rabbit patients present with gastrointestinal disease. For clinicians already working with rabbits, Dr. Reusch's article will serve as a review and for those just getting started, it will provide a comprehensive introduction into rabbit gastroenterology.

My deepest gratitude is extended to all of the authors of this issue. Their time, effort, and expertise have been eloquently captured on these pages to create a comprehensive, up-to-date text on gastroenterology in exotic companion animals. I hope all readers of this issue will be able to glean useful information from these pages that can be applied to daily clinical practice to provide the most comprehensive and progressive diagnosis of gastrointestinal disorders in their exotic animal patients.

Tracey K. Ritzman, DVM, DABVP-Avian
Avian & Exotic Animal Medicine
Angell Animal Medical Center
350 South Huntington Avenue
Boston, MA 02130, USA

E-mail address: tritzman@mspca.org

VETERINARY
CLINICS
Exotic Animal Practice

ELSEVIER
SAUNDERS

Vet Clin Exot Anim 8 (2005) 183–195

A Glimpse of the Human Field of Gastroenterology and Applications for Veterinary Medicine

Chris Griffin, DVM, DABVP-Avian[a,*],
Joseph W. Griffin Jr, MD, DABIM[b]

[a]Griffin Avian and Exotic Veterinary Hospital, 2100 Lane Street,
Kannapolis, NC 28083, USA
[b]Augusta Gastroenterology Associates, 1514 Anthony Road, Augusta,
GA 30904, USA

Welcome to a brief look at the possible future of veterinary gastroenterology. Rather than being a definitive projection of what things will be like in a few years, the following passages will instead reveal potential techniques for both diagnostic and therapeutic modalities that may become available for veterinary implementation. A definitive diagnosis is ideal, when possible, so that available treatments can be refined from general to specific therapy. As the medical profession continues its pursuit of technologic and therapeutic advancements, there is good opportunity to integrate these new practices into veterinary medicine.

Conditions such as proventricular dilation disease, Helicobacter infections, Clostridial enterotoxemia, malabsorption/maldigestion, and ileus have for years been frustrating in their diagnosis or treatment. Although there is no perfect test to diagnose or ideal protocol to treat these conditions, the advancements discussed in the following pages may very well increase the practitioner's ability to accurately determine which condition is affecting each patient. This definitive diagnosis will hopefully allow more specific therapy resulting in a quicker, more complete recovery, when possible, or more effective management of chronic disease.

Patient size, or anatomic or physiologic deviations from the more commonly studied species often limits veterinarians who treat avian and exotic patients. The airsac system in birds, for instance, makes ultrasound

---

* Corresponding author.
  E-mail address: Cgriffin7@carolina.rr.com (C. Griffin).

difficult, with much of the internal organs unavailable to standard scanning techniques. Endoscopic ultrasound (EUS), from within the lumen of the gastrointestinal (GI) tract, may very well provide a new, more complete imaging technique of the surrounding structures including liver, spleen, pancreas, mesentery, and even heart. Capsule endoscopy may eventually provide images for our larger patients that have been, up to this point, unavailable. The use of medications, including proton pump inhibitors (PPIs), new nonsteroidal anti-inflammatories, and new generations of anti-microbials may greatly increase our effectiveness in managing certain diseases. Serologic and tissue testing (for antigens, antibodies, and proteins associated with specific diseases) may help us in the diagnosis of new or existing conditions.

As much of the last 25 years has been an era of fantastic breakthroughs and advancement within veterinary medicine, and perhaps especially within avian and exotic pet medicine, the next few years will continue this trend. There surely will be more discoveries than can be alluded to in the following pages, but perhaps veterinary practitioners will witness some of these modalities come of age in the near future.

Before moving into the future of avian and exotic GI medicine, a brief review of the current status of the evaluation of GI disorders in humans is required. Clinical gastroenterologists have many tools available to evaluate the myriad of complaints related to the hollow organs of the alimentary tract. Likewise, the solid organs, liver and pancreas, can now be extensively investigated via a variety of laboratory and imaging modalities.

Most physicians rely on the patient history and physical exam to direct these investigations. Initially, acute problems are evaluated relying on standard laboratory testing such as complete blood counts, stool specimens for blood, and bacterial/fungal/viral culture. Biochemical profiles and various measurements of enzymes indicating inflammation of one or more organs are also used as part of the standard laboratory panel—transaminases, alanine aminotransferase (ALT) and aspartate aminotransferase (AST) (for suspected hepatocellular injury), alkaline phosphatase, and gamma glutamyl transpeptidase plus bilirubin (for suspected obstructive or infiltrative liver disease). Serum amylase and lipase are tested when pancreatitis is considered.

Specialty laboratory testing is used when indicated including stool antigens for giardia lamblia, stool viral studies, and stool toxins for *Clostridium difficile* and toxigenic *Escherichia coli*. Recently, a stool antigen for *Helicobacter pylori* has been shown to have excellent sensitivity and specificity. For *H pylori* diagnosis, there are also urea breath tests available; exploiting the fact that Helicobacter is a urease-producing organism. The patient ingests a urea containing solution, with carbon marked by either radioactive or other means. Twenty to 30 minutes later, the exhaled breath of the patient will contain these marked carbon particles (if suffering a Helicobacter infection), which can be detected at a reference lab via either nuclear scintigraphy or mass spectrometry.

If viral hepatitis is in the differential diagnosis, then antigens and antibodies for hepatitis A, B, and C are available, very reliable, and widely used. For persistent/chronic viral hepatitis, the viral DNA for hepatitis B and viral RNA for hepatitis C enable a documentation of active viral replication in the patient. Quantification techniques allow for determination of viral load, which is often useful to estimate a patient's chance of response to therapy and to evaluate for viral suppression and eradication. Likewise, determination of the viral genotype is also beneficial in therapeutic decision making.

There are a variety of markers for autoimmune diseases, including antinuclear antibody for chronic active hepatitis, antimitochondrial antibody for primary biliary cirrhosis, and specific enzyme determinations for disease where enzyme deficiency may be the etiology. An example of the latter would be alpha-1 antitrypsin deficiency, which may cause progressive liver and/or pulmonary disease.

Imaging of the GI tract has long used conventional contrast radiography such as barium and soluble contrast studies either by oral ingestion or rectal instillation. Gastroenterologists have heavily employed flexible fiber optic endoscopy for nearly 4 decades to directly view the esophagus, stomach, proximal small bowel, and colon. A variety of diagnostic and therapeutic techniques are routinely used through the fiber optic instruments allowing for specific diagnosis and confirmation by biopsy, tissue resection (polypectomy), injection therapy for control of bleeding, laser applications for a variety of lesions, and banding of vascular abnormalities such as esophageal varices.

Specialized techniques have been developed and widely employed for almost 30 years, allowing placement of catheters through endoscopes into the ampulla of Vater for injection of contrast to visualize both bile and pancreatic ducts (endoscopic retrograde cholangiopancreatography—ERCP). Therapeutic ERCP employs a variety of techniques including incision of the ampulla (papillotomy) to enable bile duct stone removal, for dilation of strictures, and for introduction of stents to relieve benign or malignant obstruction. Additionally, a variety of specimens including biopsies and brushings can be obtained to confirm a diagnosis of infection, malignancy, or other disease.

Another advanced application of standard endoscopy has been the technique of EUS to allow further definition of mucosal lesions, submucosal masses, wall thickness of organs, and better definition in selective instances of pancreatic masses, bile duct lesions, etc. Endoluminal ultrasound techniques have been a mainstay of various specialties including gynecology, urology, and proctology for many years to further define cysts, masses, tissue consistency/irregularities, and to allow endoscopic directed biopsies. Cardiologists for many years have routinely used transesophageal sonographic techniques known as transesophageal echocardiograms for improved assessment of posterior lying cardiac structures and cardiac function. In GI conditions, therapeutic EUS involves guided fine-needle aspirations and biopsies to confirm a diagnosis of either a benign or malignant localized lesion, such as an islet cell tumor of the pancreas, pancreatic cancer, or leiomyoma of the esophagus or stomach and other lesions.

Even with all the advancements in GI endoscopy in the last quarter of the century, and the marked improvements in imaging quality with the use of video endoscopic technology, about 75% of the 22 feet of the small intestine has remained elusive and an enigma until very recently. Standard radiographs using barium or water soluble contrast even with double contrast techniques, referred to as enteroclysis, have left much to be desired in defining vascular lesions, early small bowel tumors, small bowel inflammatory conditions, and numerous other problems. Over the past decade, a great deal of work has gone into the development of a wireless "capsule" endoscope. The history of the development of this technology is indeed fascinating, and the reader is referred to a reference on capsule endoscopy in the January 2004 Gastrointestinal Endoscopy Clinics of North America for specific details. The initial clinical experiments with the capsule were conducted in the late 1990s and reported in May of 2000 at the national Digestive Disease Week meeting in the United States. Scientific publication occurred nearly simultaneously in the journal *Nature*.

The current marketed capsule endoscope is 11 mm wide × 26 mm long and equipped with six light emitting diodes for illumination, an 8-hour battery, a semiconductor chip composed of 256 × 256 pixels, taking up to 55,000 images in the 8-hour examination (Fig. 1). The images are downloaded via a recorder, and the physician views the images at a computer workstation, generally using a 17-inch computer monitor designed to give an image of 4 inches in diameter. The capsule yields a magnification of about 1.8, which is greater than the standard endoscopic magnification. Localization of the capsule and the images (and thereby the detected abnormalities) is accomplished by strapping a series of antennas or sensors on the patient's abdomen (Fig. 2). The closest sensor receives the strongest radio-emitted signal from the capsule, and a specially developed "localization module" software package allows for both timing and relative abdominal localization of the capsule for a given set of images. Interpretation of a wireless capsule study may take 60 to 90 minutes by the physician examiner. The patient will usually pass the capsule in the feces in the next 24 to 48 hours. Occasionally, a capsule will become impacted in the area of a stricture and may be retained indefinitely. The factors influencing the decision to operate on that patient may include the nature of the stricture, symptoms of partial obstruction related to the impaction of the capsule, and bleeding. A patient of one of the authors (J.W.G.) recently passed a capsule that had been retained for 7 months, and during that time period the individual was totally asymptomatic. Progress of the capsule was followed by standard abdominal radiography.

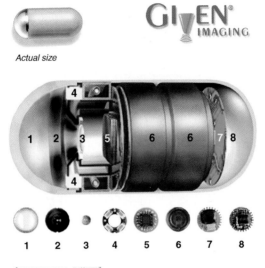

Actual size

INSIDE THE *Pillcam*

1. Optical dome
2. Lens holder
3. Lens
4. Illuminating LEDs (Light Emitting Diode)
5. CMOS (Complementary Metal Oxide Semiconductor) imager
6. Battery
7. ASIC (Application Specific Integrated Circuit) transmitter
8. Antenna

Fig. 1. Pillcam SB capsule with inside details. (*From* Given Imaging, www.givenimaging.com; with permission.)

Indications for wireless capsule endoscopic examination includes obscure GI bleeding, further evaluation of abnormal results of standard imaging studies, unexplained chronic abdominal pain, anemia, and chronic diarrhea. Small intestinal inflammatory bowel diseases, polyposis syndromes, intestinal ischemia, and drug-induced ulcerations and bleeding are all well evaluated by capsule endoscopy (Figs. 3 and 4). Erosions, ulcerations, vascular ectasias, tumors, parasites, diverticula, and a number of other lesions are readily identified (Figs. 5 and 6). Capsule endoscopy has been referred to as a novel technology, which will result in a "paradigm shift" in our capabilities with endoscopic examinations.

Radiology imaging advances have also made great strides with the newer, faster computed tomography (CT) scanners, allowing for better definition of the solid organs of the abdomen. CT-directed biopsies, drainage procedures, and other therapeutic techniques are widely employed by interventional radiologists. Additionally, CT technology is now being applied in screening for colorectal polyps and early cancers. This technology, referred to as virtual colonoscopy, may be the screening study of choice in the near future

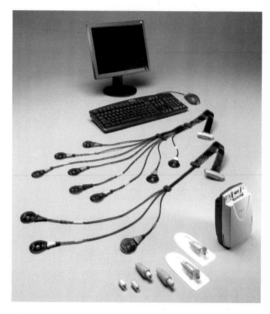

Fig. 2. Capsule endoscopy, whole system & monitor with RAPID screen. (*From* Given Imaging, www.givenimaging.com; with permission.)

in this very important area of human precancer/asymptomatic colon cancer detection.

Magnetic resonance imaging (MRI) has amazing success with the current software packages in defining bile duct and pancreatic duct abnormalities such as stones, masses, and strictures. Additionally, pancreatic lesions and vascular abnormalities, such as aneurysms, may be better defined by MRI without the need to employ iodine-containing contrasts that are potentially renal toxic. Obviously, the investment in high-speed CT scanners and state-of-the-art magnets are extraordinarily high. Use of an old radiography technique in nuclear medicine has allowed for rapid and accurate imaging of the gallbladder by radiopharmaceutical agents that are rapidly extracted by the liver and excreted into the bile. The nuclear cholangiogram/cholecysto-gram is the study of choice in a patient with suspected acute cholecystitis, either on the basis of gallstones or in the very unusual condition of acalculus cholecystitis. The addition of Doppler techniques to standard ultrasono-graphic examination allows for better definition of blood flow and char-acterization of portal hypertension, mesenteric vascular obstruction, or compromise.

Therapeutic advances in human gastroenterology have been equally important as the progress in the diagnostic realm. In the acid-related disorders of gastroesophageal reflux, stress bleeding, and peptic ulcer disease, PPIs are now the drugs of choice. Their mechanism of action is to

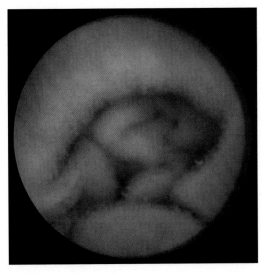

Fig. 3. Pillcam SB image of normal instestinal villi (human). (*From* Given Imaging, www.givenimaging.com; with permission.)

block the final common pathway of acid secretion in the gastric parietal cell by inhibition of the cell H+, K+, ATPase—the "proton pump." Medication is available in time-release capsules/tablets, suspensions, orally dissolving tablets, and two intravenous preparations.

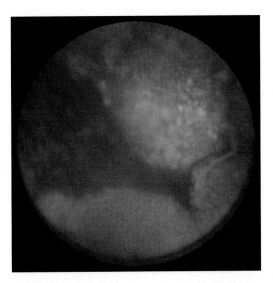

Fig. 4. Pillcam SB image of jejunum with active bleeding (human). (*From* Given Imaging, www.givenimaging.com; with permission.)

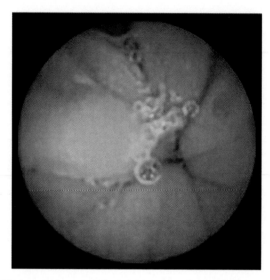

Fig. 5. Pillcam ESO image of esophagitis (human). (*From* Given Imaging, www.givenimaging. com; with permission.)

In addition to management of acid-peptic disorders, PPIs are a cornerstone in combination therapy with antibiotics for the treatment of *H pylori*. Side effects of PPIs are minimal (diarrhea, nausea) and long-term safety has now been established with over 15 years of human experience. In rats given doses from 25 to 50 times the adjusted doses based on body weight compared with humans (allometric scaling), a low incidence (1.5 to 10.0%)

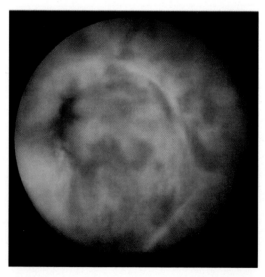

Fig. 6. Pillcam SB image of Crohn's Disease (human). (*From* Given Imaging, www.givenimaging. com; with permission.)

of enterochromaffin-like hyperplasia and enterochromaffin-like carcinoid tumors of the stomach were found. These developments have not been reported in humans.

In inflammatory bowel disorders, new developments in therapy center on the use of immunosuppressives (6-mercaptopurine, azathioprine, cyclosporine, methotrexate, and others) and biologicals, primarily antibody to tumor necrosis factor alpha (TNF). Infliximab (Remicade—Centocore) is a chimeric mouse–human antibody that effectively blocks the pro-inflammatory cytokine (TNF), but the mechanisms of action are likely multifactorial. Healing of fistulous disease in Crohn's Disease is impressive. The drug is currently given by infusion every 8 to 12 weeks. There are potential serious side effects with Infliximab including the activation of latent tuberculosis and the recent report of an increase in lymphoma in patients treated long term (1–2 years or longer).

Motility therapy has been somewhat at a standstill since the withdrawal of cisapride a few years ago, but the recent development of a serotonin antagonist and a serotonin agonist have opened new possibilities in the management of chronic diarrhea and constipation, respectively. Alosetron, marketed as Lotronex tablets (GlaxoSmithKline), is a selective antagonist of the serotonin 5-HT3 receptor and has a significant benefit in diarrhea and urgency seen in patients with irritable bowel syndrome. Side effects include constipation and a low risk of ischemic bowel problems. Tegaserod, released as Zelnorm (Novartis) tablets, is a 5-HT4 receptor agonist and has been shown to benefit patients with the constipation/bloating form of irritable bowel syndrome. Zelnorm is being investigated as a therapy for various forms of ileus. The major side effects are typically diarrhea and abdominal cramping, often occurring early after the initiation of treatment.

In humans, probiotics are gaining more widespread use in several conditions including antibiotic associated diarrhea, pouchitis (inflammation of the surgically formed ileal pouch following proctocolectomy for chronic ulcerative colitis), and in chronic diarrhea of unknown etiology. A new, nonsystemic antibiotic, rifaximin (Xifaxan – Salix), is now available in the United States to treat traveler's diarrhea caused by noninvasive strains of E coli, one of the most common causes of diarrhea in international travelers.

This clearly is not an exhaustive and complete review of all techniques for unraveling the many mysteries of conditions inside the abdomen. Hopefully, it has been a brief but illuminating review. These advancements may have direct application in the progression of avian and exotic pet medicine. A few examples follow, but there are an infinite number of creative ways to implement this newer technology.

Avian

Avian patients present many challenges for the practitioner in the diagnosis and treatment of GI disorders. Their small size (some pet birds weigh less than 20 g) and the presence of the air sac system make direct (nonradiographic) imaging difficult. Ultrasound examination, while becoming more widely used, still faces the problems associated with an air-filled cavity. The use of EUS to evaluate the esophagus, crop, proventriculus, ventriculus, and upper small intestine may provide a fresh look and new information, particularly when there are thickenings within the intestinal tract.

Examining other internal organs, including liver, heart, pancreas, spleen, gonads, and kidneys via this technique may also result in new information about both normal and abnormal tissue, and may help to solve some of the mysteries associated with diseases of these systems. Some of these organs, particularly the kidneys, adrenals, and possibly gonads, may be accessible from a cloacal approach, while the others may be accessible from an orad approach. Of great interest, although outside the scope of this topic, is the possible use of transesophageal ultrasound to evaluate the heart of our avian patients. The technology that will allow us to proceed with these techniques is continuing to evolve, and hopefully there will be ultrasound probes of appropriate size available in the near future.

The endoscope appears to be the most versatile tool for diagnostic applications in avian patients. Advances made in cloacoscopy by Dr. Taylor, among others, and initial techniques perfected by Drs. Harris, Taylor, Murray, and others, make rigid endoscopy an extremely flexible tool for veterinary use. Augmenting its capacity for gathering information by adding the possibility of ultrasound examinations may continue the field's progression toward the highest levels of medicine.

Capsule endoscopy may also be a viable technology within the next decade. The size of the capsule, currently about 1 by 2.5 cm, makes it problematic to pass in all but the largest birds. A smaller capsule may become available over the next several years, and that would be very helpful. Also, the positioning of the receptor probes may be problematic, as many parrots would resist this type of invasion. It would not take long for a cockatoo to destroy the (probably expensive) receptors if it chose to do so. However, there is still legitimate potential use for this technology, from helping to diagnose motility disorders (a look inside the poorly contracting proventriculus and ventriculus) to allowing for visual confirmation of inflammation, ulceration, stricture, or even foreign bodies.

Continued research into testing for toxins produced by pathogenic microbes (bacterial or fungal) within the human field may lead to similar testing becoming readily available for veterinary use. Fecal screening for toxins associated with *Clostridium* sp, *E coli*, and *Aspergillus* sp may provide quick diagnosis for these conditions, leading to quicker and more appropriately directed medical therapy. There are understood differences between human pathogens and avian (and other animal) pathogens, but in many cases, there is significant conservation of DNA or protein sequences that may allow for minimal alterations in the testing procedures. Some of these tests are, in all likelihood, being developed for the veterinary field at this time.

As for other systematic evaluations of motility, other techniques, not discussed here in depth, may become more available as this technology progresses in the coming years. Real-time CT scans and MRIs (with or without contrast) may provide better images and more effective quantification of peristalsis in our avian patients than fluoroscopy, which is currently being used at a few select locations in North America. Also, the progression of anti-inflammatory research and development may provide even more effective medications for treating conditions like proventricular dilatation disease, which currently is managed with drugs like meloxicam and celocoxib.

Rabbits and other hindgut fermenting mammals

For rabbits and guinea pigs, among others, ileus is still one of the most common and difficult presentations for veterinarians. Although the syndrome is well known, and general supportive care is effective in many of the cases, more specific therapy may be available for these patients if diagnosis of the underlying cause(s) can be more readily accomplished. Stress often plays a role in ileus, and bacterial overgrowth (sometimes *Clostridium* sp or others) can be a complicating factor. Tests that reveal the presence of toxins produced by specific bacteria may more quickly and accurately diagnose a condition than some stains (including Gram stains) and bacterial cultures, which rely on the presence of the bacteria in a sample for diagnosis. Quicker and more accurate diagnosis would allow for quicker and more precise treatment as well. The use of implanted peristaltic pacemakers in people is in its infancy, and this technique may eventually be helpful for our rabbit (or guinea pig) patients suffering from ileus.

The thin-wall structure and friable nature of the rabbit colon and cecum make colonoscopy a risky procedure in these pets. However, continued use of imaging for oral procedures as is commonly done for oral examinations and dental work, may lead to more commonly employed upper GI endoscopy to help visualize the stomach and the contents within. Perhaps techniques will continue to be developed that may help to break up gastric foreign bodies containing fiber and aid in the treatment of GI stasis (when stomach foreign bodies are part of that multifactorial syndrome).

Ferrets

Ferrets present multiple challenges for the practitioner, from their wiggly nature to their manifold illnesses. Tests for Helicobacter identification have been discussed for several years, and hopefully will become more widely available in the near future. Other testing, including the stool antigen tests and various urea breath tests used in humans, may provide more tools to help in the diagnosis of Helicobacter infections. Therapy for Helicobacter should be directed toward treatment with appropriate antibiotics (metronidazole and either amoxicillin, clarithromycin, or a cephalosporin), changing the acid levels and pH with H-2 blockers or PPIs, and using bismuth subsalicylate, which is known to be effective against Helicobacter.

Upper GI endoscopy can be used in the ferret for stomach biopsies, although the ease of standard laparotomy and gastrotomy may preclude the development of this procedure. However, the magnification provided by endoscopic examination may allow for more directed biopsy site determination. Capsule endoscopy and endoscopic-assisted ultrasound may also provide benefits, for many of the same reasons listed above in the avian section. Esophageal echocardiography may help to reveal masses or other problems outside of the GI tract.

Reptiles

It would seem that the snake is the perfect candidate for endoscopic evaluation. The basic linear nature of the reptile GI tract can be taken advantage of once the snake patient reaches a certain size. The long nature of the snake trachea may also allow for examination via rigid or flexible endoscopy, although methods to allow for oxygenation and perfusion (perhaps similar to placement of an airsac tube in birds) may need to be further developed to allow for lengthy (time-wise) examinations.

The relatively simple structure of the reptile GI tract has been amenable to the standard surgical approaches and techniques when needed. Research and development is continuing in the sectors of diagnostics and treatments for such diseases as Inclusion Body Disease of Boids, paramyxovirus infections, cryptosporidia infections, and others. The hope is that these new developments will become available in forms that will allow more in hospital use. Advances in DNA sequencing and other technologies will push the progression with increasing velocity in the coming years.

Newer techniques used routinely by some referral institutions such as iguana cystoscopy and endoscopic ovariohysterectomy will become more refined, and through seminars and laboratories disseminated to the more general exotic pet practitioners.

For a more complete review of the current status of gastroenterology within exotic veterinary medicine, please see the rest of this volume of *Veterinary Clinics of North America Exotic Animal Practice* and the items listed in the suggested reading list found at the end of this article.

In summary, it has been the purpose of the preceding pages to spark creative ideas to push the veterinary profession forward in the coming years. Refined endoscopic techniques, advances in antigen, antibody, and toxin detection, improved imaging techniques, and next generation medications will provide the means, but only as far as the profession itself can creatively and effectively use these tools. Veterinary practitioners, especially those in the field of avian, reptile, and exotic mammal medicine, must be innovative and think outside the box, on top of the box, within the box, and then must investigate whether the box itself needs to be redefined and recognized as something both well studied and unknown. The path to the future is easy enough, but where it takes us will be the results of innovation, effort, ingenuity, and insight.

Suggested reading

Altman RB, Clubb SL, Dorrenstein GM, et al, editors. Avian medicine and surgery. Philadelphia: WB Saunders; 1997. p. 412–53.

Barkin JS, editor. Wireless capsule endoscopy. Gastrointest Endosc Clin North Am 2004;14(1).

Fudge AM, editor. Laboratory medicine avian and exotic pets. Philadelphia: WB Saunders; 2000.

Hara AK, Leighton JA, Sharma VK, et al. Small bowel: preliminary comparison of capsule endoscopy with barium study and CT. Radiology 2004;230(1):260–5 [Epub 2003 Nov 14].

Hawes RH. Endoscopic ultrasound. Gastrointest Endosc Clin North Am 2000;10:161–74.

Kimmey MB, editor. The NIH state-of-the-science conference: ERCP for diagnosis and therapy. Gastrointest Endosc 2002;56:S153–302.

Mader DR, editor. Reptile medicine and surgery. Philadelphia: WB Saunders; 1996.

McArthur S, Wilkinson R, Meyer J, editors. Medicine and surgery of tortoises and turtles. Ames (IA): Blackwell Publishing; 2003.

Mow WS, Lo SL, Targon SR, et al. Initial experience with wireless capsule enteroscopy in diagnosis and management of inflammatory bowel disease. Clin Gastroenterol Hepatol 2004;2:31–40.

Nguyen MT. Abnormal liver function tests. In: Edmundowickz SA, editor. Common problems in gastroenterology. New York: McGraw–Hill Medical Publishing Division; 2002. p. 271–85.

Pennazio M, Santucci R, Rondonotti E, et al. Outcome of patients with obscure gastrointestinal bleeding after capsule endoscopy: report of 100 consecutive cases. Gastroenterology 2004; 126(3):643–53.

Quesenberry KE, Carpenter JW, editors. Ferrets, rabbits and rodents clinical medicine and surgery. St. Louis (MO): Saunders; 2002.

Ritchie BW, Harrison GJ, Harrison LR, editors. Avian medicine: principles and application. Lake Worth (FL): Wingers Publishing; 1994. p. 223–61; 482–521.

Rupley AE, editor. Manual of avian practice. Philadelphia: WB Saunders; 1997. p. 91–133.

Rupley AE, editor. Veterinary clinics of North America exotic animal practice, therapeutics, Vol. 3. Philadelphia: WB Saunders; 2000.

Rupley AE, editor. Veterinary clinics of North America exotic animal practice, internal medicine, Vol. 6. Philadelphia: WB Saunders; 2003.

ELSEVIER
SAUNDERS

VETERINARY
CLINICS
Exotic Animal Practice

Vet Clin Exot Anim 8 (2005) 197–212

The Ferret Gastrointestinal Tract and *Helicobacter mustelae* Infection

Cathy A. Johnson-Delaney, DVM, DABVP[a,b,c,*]

[a]*Avian and Exotics Advanced Diagnostic Consulting, c/o Exotic Pet & Bird Clinic,*
903 5th Avenue, Suite 101, Kirkland, WA 98033, USA
[b]*Exotic Pet & Bird Clinic, 903 5th Avenue, Suite 101, Kirkland, WA 98033, USA*
[c]*Bird and Exotic Clinic of Seattle, 4019 Aurora Avenue N, Seattle, WA 98103, USA*

The gastrointestinal tract of the domestic ferret, *Mustela putorius furo*, has been studied extensively as a model for several human gastrointestinal tract diseases, including spontaneous gastric and duodenal ulcers, gastroesophageal reflux, gastric carcinoma and lymphoma, the lack of acid mucosubstances similar to humans, and *Helicobacter mustelae* infection. To discuss the implications of the role of *Helicobacter* in disease, we must first review the unique anatomy and physiology of the ferret digestive system.

Physiologically hypermotile and secretory

The ferret has a short gastrointestinal transit time, 148 to 219 minutes when fed a meat-based diet. The digestive system is under vagal and sacral innervation. The tract is spontaneously active even under anesthesia. Motility can be moderated with atropine. The stomach spontaneously produces acids and proteolytic enzymes. Histamine and vagal stimulation provoke more secretions [1].

Gut closure for antibody absorption occurs in kits between 28 and 42 days of age. Ferrets can absorb beta carotene and convert it to retinoic acid. Carbohydrases and proteolytic activity take place distally in the jejunum rather than more proximally in the duodenum [1].

* Avian and Exotics Advanced Diagnostic Consulting, c/o Exotic Pet & Bird Clinic, 903 5th Avenue, Suite 101, Kirkland, WA 98033, USA.
E-mail address: cajddvm@hotmail.com

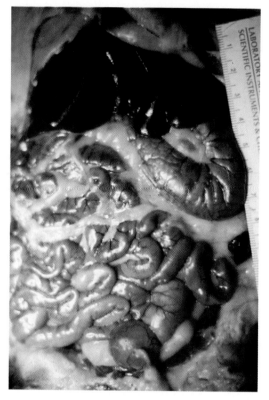

Fig. 1. Ferret stomach and intestinal tract in situ. Note prominent vascularity of stomach and enlarged lymph node in the fat of the lesser curvature. This ferret was subsequently diagnosed with *H mustelae* gastritis.

The stomach

The ferret has a simple stomach, similar in shape to that of the dog. Fig. 1 shows a ferret stomach and intestinal tract in situ. Note the prominent vasculature of the stomach as well as the prominent lymph node lying in the lesser curvature. This was a confirmed case of *H mustelae* gastritis upon histopathology. It is innervated by parasympathetic fibers from the vagus nerve and sympathetic fibers via the celiacomesenteric plexus. The stomach has considerable storage capacity (100 mL of milk in 10 minutes in an adult). Eighty percent of a meal is stored in the proximal stomach [1].

The lower esophageal sphincter (LES) and the mechanisms of gastro-esophageal reflux in the ferret are being used as an animal model [2,3] Transient LES relaxation is the mechanism, and is unassociated with swallowing in the ferret just as in humans [4]. Gastric infusions of glucose, lipid, and gas are all effective in provoking gastroesophageal reflux in the ferret. Lipid and glucose stimulated acid secretion [4]. The fundus of the stomach and the LES are coinnervated by vagal preganglionic motor neurons, as these sections work in tandem: the LES must relax to accommodate food during ingestion or preceding emesis. The antrum of the stomach provides mixing and propulsion of contents for gastric emptying and are innervated by neurons responding to differing neurotransmitters [5–9]. The ferret is used as an emetic model to test antiemetics. Serotonin successfully blocks cisplatin at 10 mg/kg induced emesis [10]. An antiemetic pursued in the ferret model has been delta9-tetrahydrocannabinol (Δ^9-THC), the cannabinoid that is antiemetic in humans. Ferrets have the Cannabinoid1 receptor in the dorsal motor vagal nucleus, with cell bodies in the area postrema, nucleus tractus solitarius, and nodose ganglion. This receptor mediates the antiemetic action of cannabinoids [11,12]. Δ^9-THC was found to cause gastroesophageal reflux due to the relaxation of the lower esophageal sphincter. This effect may have implications in the treatment of gastroesophageal reflux and other upper gastrointestinal disorders [12].

The ferret stomach also secretes acid in response to histamine, pentagastrin, and calcium. There is a low concentration of free histamine in the stomach. The ferret lacks the histamine-forming enzyme (L-histidine decarboxylase) in the stomach, although histamine-destroying activity is present. Histamine also stimulates secretion of proteolytic enzymes. Histamine H2 receptor antagonists abolish the acid secretion response to exogenous histamine or exogenous stimulation with pentagastrin. Atropine only reduces acid secretion by 30% [1].

Gastrin is secreted in the gastric antrum and duodenum. Hypoglycemia induced by insulin produces a sustained stimulation of acid secretion [1]. This is particularly relevant to ferrets with insulinomas: therapy needs to include medications that decrease acid secretion.

The intestine

The ferret intestine consists of three sections. Villi and goblet cells are present in all sections. The duodenum is the proximal segment. The duodenum is innervated by vagal preganglionic parasympathic neurons originating in the dorsal motor nucleus of the vagal nerve in the brainstem [13]. The major duodenal papilla contains the common opening for the bile and pancreatic ducts. This is located about 3 cm from the pylorus. The minor papilla may be absent. Brunner's glands are present in the submucosa of duodenum proximal to bile duct. The glands produce only neutral mucosubstances as in humans [1].

The jejunal and ileal segments cannot be distinguished, and may be referred to as the "jejunoileum," which ends at the ascending colon. The small intestine is innervated by the vagus nerve and the sympathetic trunks arise from the celiac and cranial mesenteric plexus [1].

Motility is affected by the hormones secretin, pancreozymin-cholecysto-kinin(PZ-CCK), an unidentified vasoconstrictor, vasoactive intestinal polypeptide (VIP), and substance P. VIP inhibits jejunal motor activity due to vagal simulation while substance P excites activity. Both increase water secretion by jejunal epithelium. The muscular layer has a higher concentration of these hormones than the epithelium. Jejunal motility mediated by hormones is not blocked by atropine. 5-hydroxytryptamine (5-HT$_3$) and synthetic serotonin receptor agonists induce large contraction and defecation. The basal colonic motility pattern was not changed, and the large contractions can be blocked with a receptor antagonist. The implications of this model are for testing pharmaceuticals for constipation without undesired changes in gut motility patterns [14]. Cervical (mechanical) vagus stimulation will affect motility. This has significant implications for the clinician, who during intubation, may manipulate the neck and thorax and inadvertently stimulate the vagus nerve and stimulate intestinal motility at the beginning of surgery.

The large intestine is composed of the colon and rectum. There is no cecum and no ileocolic junction. The junction is inferred by the presence of the anastomoses of the jejunal artery with the ileocolic artery. The colon consists of the ascending, transverse, and descending colon, with the largest being the decending. The colon is innervated by autonomic fibers from the vagus, cranial, and caudal mesenteric plexus [1].

There are tubular glands and goblet cells in the colon. These secrete sulfated mucosubstances. The motility of the colon resembles that of a dog ileum. Motility is vagus-dependent and mediated by cholinergic and noncholinergic fibers. Sacral innervation is excitatory. Retroperistalsis begins in the colon that may be the genesis of vomiting in the ferret [1].

Exocrine pancreas and biliary system

The exocrine pancreas and biliary system are also under vagal stimulation. There is a trophic relationship with capillary connections between the islets and the exocrine pancreatic tissue. A bile salt-dependent lipase is produced. The adult jill mammary tissue is high in this enzyme. Ferret milk has lipase activity 10 to 20 times higher than human milk. If lipase elevations are present in the blood, consider pancreatic inflammation or disease [1].

The gallbladder contracts in response to cholecystokinin. Cholecystokinin is found throughout the gastrointestinal tract. This contraction inhibits gastric emptying and stimulates small intestine and colonic motility. The contractile response directly affects smooth muscles or neurons, which furthers intestinal motility [1].

In summary, the ferret gastrointestinal tract is designed to be excitatory, have rapid motility, and be highly secretory. Exogenous stressors, chemical and neurologic stimulations, further increase motility and secretion. During any hypoglycemic episode the clinician needs to be aware of the pancreatic and gastric physiology and treat the nausea and secretions in addition to the hypoglycemia. It may also be prudent to administer medication to inhibit acid secretions before surgeries and in any stressed or ill ferrets.

The role of *Helicobacter mustelae* in gastrointestinal disease

H mustelae was originally isolated from gastric tissue of one ferret with a gastric ulcer and from two ferrets with normal gastric mucosa [15]. The ferret organism was morphologically and biochemically similar to *Helicobacter pylori*, but DNA relatedness and 16S rRNA sequence analyses proved that it was a novel species [15]. Nomenclature was changed from Campylobacter-like (*C mustelae*) which still appears in the older literature. *H mustelae* infection in ferrets remains the best-studied animal model of gastric *Helicobacter* in its natural host and provides the opportunity to study the relationship between infection and disease [15].

H mustelae is a small rod (0.5 × 2 μm), sometimes slightly curved, with multiple sheathed flagella located at both poles as well as laterally. Fig. 2 illustrates *H mustelae* in ferret gastric mucosa stained with Warthin-Starry stain. Like other species of gastric *Helicobacter*, *H mustelae* hydrolyzes urea, although it is distinctive due to susceptibility to nalidixic acid. The fatty acid composition and protein profiles are distinct from *H pylori*, the human gastric *Helicobacter* [15]. Phylogenetically it is closer to *Helicobacter* species that infect the colon or hepatobiliary systems of other animal species [15]. Unlike *H pylori*, which has considerable heterogeneity unless derived from the same or related persons, *H mustelae* genome is highly conserved [15]. The author speculates that this may be because the domesticated ferret is highly inbred, and most ferrets used for these studies came from one breeding farm.

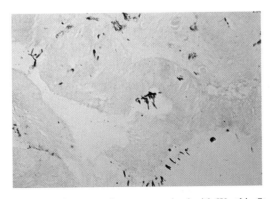

Fig. 2. *H mustelae* in ferret gastric mucosa stained with Warthin-Starry stain.

Epizootiology

Studies have shown that the prevalence of *H mustelae* infection increases with age. In kits less than 1 month of age it is not present, but by 1 year of age 100% are infected [15]. It has been found in ferrets worldwide, and can be considered a member of the resident flora of the ferret stomach [15].

Transmission

Fox and colleagues suggest that transmission of *H mustelae* occurs via the fecal–oral route and is promoted by hypochlorhydria [15–17]. Increased gastric pH permits bacteria to exit the stomach and enter the lower gastrointestinal tract, where they can be recovered in feces. This may provide the mechanism for transmission. Adult chronically infected ferrets treated with a proton pump inhibitor (omeprazole) had a rise in gastric pH, and recovery of *H mustelae* in fecal cultures was increased compared with that before treatment [15].

Disease

Naturally infected ferrets have a predominantly mononuclear gastritis composed of lymphocytes and plasma cells, with only occasional eosinophilic and polymorphonuclear leukocytes [15]. In the corpus of the ferret stomach, gastritis is mononuclear, minimal, or superficially in the mucosa. The bacteria predominate in the antrum where the inflammatory infiltrate can occupy the full thickness of the mucosa including the gastric pit, portions of the glands, and the mucosal surface. This is similar to the diffuse antral gastritis seen in humans infected with *H pylori* [15]. Infected ferrets produce elevated immunoglobulin G (IgG) titers to *H mustelae*. Ferrets also generate autoantibodies to gastric parietal cells [18]. Koch's postulate has been confirmed by administration of the organism to specific

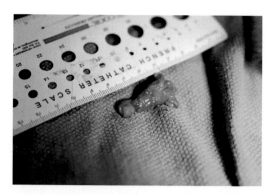

Fig. 3. Pylorus with mucosal ulceration. *Helicobacter* was identified on histopathology.

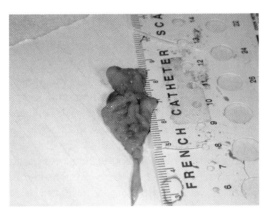

Fig. 4. Hemorrhagic erosions within the gastric mucosa of a ferret with *H mustelae* gastritis.

pathogen free for *H mustelae* developed gastric colonization, chronic gastritis, and elevation of serum anti-*H mustelae* antibody titer [19]. Infection is life-long, and the severity of the gastritis increases with age [19].

Ferrets develop gastric ulcers and hemorrhagic gastric erosions (35% in one group of 31 ferrets in England) but it was not demonstrated that *H mustelae* was the cause of peptic ulcer disease although it can occasionally be seen in ferrets with gastric ulcers [15]. Fig. 3 shows the pylorus of a ferret with a large ulcer. Fig. 4 shows hemorrhagic erosions within gastric mucosa of a ferret. Fig. 5 shows the histopathology of a gastric ulcer. *H mustelae*-infected ferrets may develop duodenal ulcer or gastric ulcer, with the latter associated with atrophic gastritis, dysplasia, and gastric adenocarcinoma. This model mimics the relationship between human hosts and infection with *H pylori*. Hypergastrinemia, which is a feature of humans infected with *H pylori* and associated with duodenal ulcerative disease, has also been documented in the ferret [19].

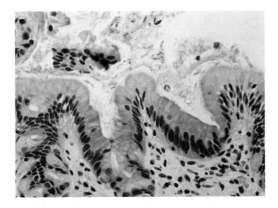

Fig. 5. Histopathology of a ferret gastric ulcer.

The role of *H mustelae* in gastric tumors of the ferret has not been clearly demonstrated. Gastric adenocarcinoma and gastric mucosa-associated lymphoid tissue lymphoma have occasionally been found in the ferret in association with *H mustelae* [15,20,21]. Uninfected ferret stomachs are devoid of lymphoid follicles. When naturally infected as weanlings, ferrets develop lymphoproliferation, which increases in extent and severity. Chronically infected ferrets appear to be at increased risk of developing gastric lymphomas in the wall of the lesser curvature of the pyloric antrum. This is the predominant location of *H mustelae*-induced gastritis in ferrets [19].

Hepatobiliary inflammation and hepatic hemangiosarcomas have been diagnosed in ferrets. In these ferrets, there was chronic colangiohepatitis with cellular proliferation ranging from hyperplasia to carcinoma. The *Helicobacter* species were sequenced and had 98% and 97% similarity to *Helicobacter cholecystus* and *Helicobacter* sp strain 266-11, respectively [22]. The role of *Helicobacter* species in hepatitis or hepatic neoplasia requires further study [22].

Helicobacter sp is being investigated for its role in inflammatory bowel disease, ulcerative colitis, and colonic adenocarcinoma in other animal models such as the mouse and the cotton-top tamarin [23,24]. *Helicobacter* sp has been found in association with ulcerative colitis in humans [25]. *H cinaedi* has been isolated from the inflamed liver and intestine of a rhesus macaque with clinically debilitating, idiopathic colitis [24]. Recent studies in mice have looked at gene dysregulation caused by helicobacter infections that occur in the absence of clinical and histologic disease. The measurement of the expression level of these key genes may be useful in assessing host response to subclinical infection. The studies found coinfection with *H rodentium* and *H hepaticus* caused significant increases in expression of the immune-regulatory gene interleukin 10, proinflammatory genes interferon gamma (IFN-γ), IFN-γ-inducible protein of 10 kDa, and macrophage inflammatory protein 1α. Clinical disease was seen in immunomodified mice (scid/Trp53$-/-$) that have the null mutation for the p53 tumor suppressor gene. The disease included hemorrhagic diarrhea, proliferative typhlocolitis, and cholangiohepatitis [26]. It has been speculated by the author that ferrets may have aberrations with one or more tumor suppressor genes. The ferret's response to infection with *Helicobacter* may be further explained through examination of the genome and enteric immune responses. Research is currently underway to explore this possibility. An enterohepatic *Helicobacter* sp has been found in some human patients with inflammatory bowel disease [27]. The role of *Helicobacter* in inflammatory bowel disease in ferrets is unknown at this time.

Diagnosis

Samples may be obtained by gastric endoscopic biopsy for microbiology and histology. Culturing the organism requires procedures not commonly

Table 1

Comparison of sample sites and techniques in diagnostic testing for *H mustelae*

Animal number	Tested by immunostaining				Tested by PCR			
	Blood	Rectal swab	Gastric swab	Tissue	Blood	Rectal swab	Gastric swab	Tissue
1	Neg	Neg	Neg	ND	LLP	LLP	+	ND
2	Neg	Neg	Neg	ND	LLP	Neg	+	ND
3	Neg	Neg	Neg	ND	Neg	Neg	Neg	ND
4	Neg	Neg	Neg	ND	Neg	Neg	Neg	ND
5	Neg	Neg	+	ND	Neg	Neg	+	ND
6	Neg	Neg	Neg	ND	Neg	+	+	ND
7	Neg	Neg	Neg	ND	Neg	Neg	+	ND
8	Neg	Neg	Neg	+	Neg	Neg	Neg	+
9	ND	ND	Neg	ND	ND	ND	Neg	ND
10	ND	ND	ND	+	ND	ND	ND	+
11	ND	ND	ND	+	ND	ND	ND	+
12	ND	ND	Neg	ND	ND	ND	Neg	ND
13	ND	ND	+	ND	ND	ND	Neg	ND
14	ND	Neg	Neg	ND	ND	Neg	+	ND
15	ND	Neg	Neg	ND	ND	Neg	Neg	ND
16	Neg	Neg	Neg	ND	Neg	Neg	+	ND
17	Neg	Neg	Neg	ND	LLP	LLP	+	ND
18	Neg	Neg	Neg	ND	Neg	Neg	+	ND
19	ND	Neg	Neg	ND	ND	Neg	LLP	ND
20	ND	Neg	Neg	ND	ND	LLP	LLP	ND
21	ND	ND	ND	ND	ND	Neg	Neg	ND
22	ND	ND	ND	ND	ND	+	Neg	ND
23	ND	ND	ND	ND	ND	+	+	ND
24	ND	ND	ND	ND	ND	Neg	Neg	ND
25	ND	ND	ND	ND	ND	Neg	+	ND
26	ND	ND	ND	ND	ND	Neg	+	ND
27	ND	ND	ND	ND	ND	LLP	Neg	ND
28	ND	ND	ND	ND	ND	+	Neg	ND
29	ND	ND	ND	ND	ND	Neg	Neg	ND
30	ND	ND	ND	ND	ND	Neg	Neg	ND
A	Neg	Neg	+	ND	Neg	LLP	+	ND
B	Neg	Neg	+	ND	Neg	Neg	+	ND
C	Neg	Neg	+	ND	Neg	Neg	+	ND
D	Neg	Neg	+	ND	Neg	Neg	+	ND
E	Neg	Neg	+	ND	Neg	Neg	+	ND
F	Neg	Neg	Neg	ND	Neg	Neg	+	ND
G	ND	Neg	Neg	ND	ND	Neg	+	ND
H	ND	Neg	ND	ND	ND	+	ND	ND
40	ND	ND	ND	ND	ND	ND	+	ND
60	ND	ND	ND	ND	ND	ND	+, + Oral	ND

Blood samples were submitted as whole blood in EDTA. Rectal and gastric swabs were collected as described in above text. Tissues were collected in 10% formalin. Testing performed by immunostaining was confirmed by histopathology. Statistical analysis and correlation with clinical disease is not represented in this table. Ferrets 41–59 were not part of this phase of data collection.

Abbreviations: ND, not done; LLP, low level positive; PCR, polymerase chain reaction.

done at veterinary diagnostic laboratories, but many human microbiology laboratories may be able to process a ferret sample. Biopsy samples can also be assayed for urease, although this assay lacks specificity and sensitivity. Intestinal reflux and blood can cause false-positive reactions. Low-level infections may not produce a demonstrable color change. Biopsy samples for histopathology should be placed into cassettes and oriented with a 25-gauge needle so that they are cut perpendicular to the plane of the mucosal surface. The Warthin-Starry and H&E stains are used for assessment of colonization and mucosal histopathologic morphology, respectively [19].

Serum antibody titers can be done although serum antibody to *H mustelae* is not protective because ferrets with high titers are already colonized by the organism and have associated gastritis. ELISA titers also rise with age and chronicity of infection. Fox has demonstrated decreasing serum titers in ferrets after eradication of *H mustelae* [19].

H mustelae can be cultured from feces. There is also a urea breath test adapted from the common human test for *H pylori*. This requires ferrets to be administered $_{14}C$ labeled urea and placed in a sealed glass metabolism chamber. Recovered $_{14}CO^2$ is measured by beta scintillation counts. This is not a practical test except in research institutions [19].

Real-time polymerase chain reaction (PCR) [Research Associates Laboratory, R.A.L., Inc., Dallas, Texas, www.vetdna.com] has now become available. This test can confirm the presence of *H mustelae* DNA, but also provides the practitioner data on the amount of organism present [28]. Immunohistochemical staining to demonstrate the presence of *Helicobacter* organisms in biopsy samples, gastric, and fecal swabs is also available to the practitioner (Research Associates Laboratory). This test can also be used following a treatment regimen to determine effectiveness of the treatment. Table 1 compares samples used in immunohistochemistry and PCR to develop a reliable commercial test for *H mustelae*. Samples were submitted by the author and Dr. Angela Lennox for development of a testing method. Results of this study show that out of 40 ferrets sampled, 23 were positive

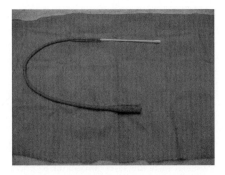

Fig. 6. Culture swab using a red rubber tube. (Courtesy of Dr. Angela Lennox.)

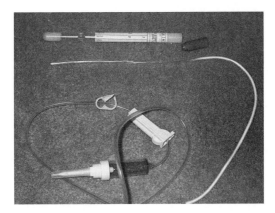

Fig. 7. Culture swab using sterile tubing cut from infusion set tubing.

for *H mustelae* on gastric swab PCR. An additional four were positive by PCR on rectal swab, although negative on other samples. Three ferrets tested positive on tissue samples by both immunostaining and PCR while negative on other tests. Only one ferret was positive on a gastric swab immunostain test while negative on all others. Thirty-three of 40 ferrets were considered positive for *H mustelae* in this trial (78%). The gastric swab PCR alone showed 74% of those positive. With this result, it would be suggested that clinicians consider submitting swabs from multiple sites (oral mucosa as shown in Table 4, stomach, and rectum).

Collection of the gastric swab for either immunohistochemical staining or PCR is relatively simple. Because standard swabs are not long enough to reach the ferret stomach, the culturette can be inserted snugly into the distal end of a soft red rubber feeding tube or a measured length of infusion set tubing, and gently passed into the stomach of a sedated ferret [28,29].

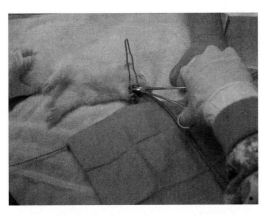

Fig. 8. Placement and technique for obtaining a gastric mucosal swab in the sedated ferret. (Courtesy of Dr. Angela Lennox.)

Table 2
Treatment regimens based on clinical trials

Effective combinations	Unsuccessful medications
Amoxicillin (30 mg/kg q 8 h × 21–28 d); metronidazole (20 mg/kg q 8 h × 21–28 d); bismuth subsalicylate (7.5 mg/kg q 8 h × 21–28 d)	Amoxicillin alone. May not be effective at q 12 h even in combinations
	Metronidazole alone. May not be effective with Amoxicillin if given at 12-h intervals
	Chloramphenicol alone
	Enrofloxacin alone
Enrofloxacin (8.5 mg/kg/day divided q 12 h × 14 d); bismuth subcitrate[a] (12 mg/kg divided q 12 h × 14 d)	Tetracycline
	Bismuth subsalicylate alone
Clarithromycin (12.5 mg/kg q 12 h × 14 d); ranitidine bismuth citrate[a] (24 mg/kg q 12 h × 14 d)	Omeprazole and amoxicillin
	Omeprazole alone
Clarithromycin (12.5 mg/kg q 8 h × 14 d); ranitidine bismuth citrate[a] (24 mg/kg q 8 h × 14 d) This is also a published dosage	

Amoxicillin: Amoxil, GlaxoSmithKline, Research Triangle Park, NC.
Metronidazole USP, Watson Laboratories, Inc., Corona, CA.
Bismuth subsalicylate: Pepto-Bismol, Proctor & Gamble, Cinncinati, OH.
Enrofloxacin: Baytril, Bayer, West Haven, CT.
Clarithromycin: Biaxin, Abbott Laboratories, Abbott Park, IL.
Omeprazole: Prilosec, AstraZeneca Pharmaceuticals LP, Wilmington, DE.
[a] not commercially available in the US.
Data from Refs. [19,28,30,31].

Intubation is advisable if the ferret has lost the swallow reflex. The stomach is gently manipulated externally to allow rubbing contact between the swab and gastric mucosa. Samples can be submitted to Research Associates Laboratory in standard bacterial culture media. Figs. 6 and 7 show swabs

Table 3
Medications used as adjunctive therapy

Drug	Dosage	Comments
Famotidine	0.25–0.5 mg/kg po, im, iv q 24 h	Histamine antagonist; available over the counter; decreases gastric acid; provides pain relief
Omeprazole	0.7 mg/kg po q 24 h	Protein pump inhibitor, short term usage only
Ranitidine USP	24 mg/kg po q 8h ×14 d	Histamine inhibitor; decreases gastric acid; provides pain relief. Tablet form available over the counter
Sucralfate	25 mg/kg po q 8 h	Coats esophageal and gastric mucosa, local effect only. Syrup palatable

Famotidine: Famotidine tablets USP, Zenith Goldine Pharmaceuticals, Inc., Miami, FL.
Omeprazole: Prilosec, AstraZeneca Pharmaceuticals LP, Wilmington, DE.
Ranitidine USP: Ranitidine Tablet USP, Perrigo Co., Allegan, MI.
Sucralfate: Carafate, Aventis Pharmaceuticals, Inc., Kansas City, MO.
Data from Refs. [28,30,32].

Table 4
Effectiveness of two treatment regimens monitored by oral and/or gastric swab polymerase chain reaction

Helicobacter swab results posttreatment

Animal number	PCR oral swab	PCR gastric swab	Days posttreatment of sample	Treatment regimen:[a]
32 Household 1	ND	Strong +++	14 d	Enroflox/metro/pepto
33	ND	Very weak +	14 d	Enroflox/metro/pepto
34	ND	Neg	14 d	Enroflox/metro/pepto
35	ND	Neg	14 d	Enroflox/metro/pepto
36	ND	Neg	14 d	Enroflox/metro/pepto
41	ND	Neg	14 d	Enroflox/metro/pepto
42	ND	Neg	14 d	Enroflox/metro/pepto
43	ND	Neg	14 d	Enroflox/metro/pepto
44	ND	Neg	14 d	Enroflox/metro/pepto
45	ND	Neg	14 d	Enroflox/metro/pepto
63	Low +	Low +	60 d	Enroflox/metro/pepto
64	Neg	Neg	60 d	Enroflox/metro/pepto
65	+	+	60 d	Enroflox/metro/pepto
52 Household 2	Neg	+	14 d	Amoxi/metro/pepto
53	Neg	Neg	14 d	Amoxi/metro/pepto
54	+	+	14 d	Amoxi/metro/pepto
55	+	Neg	14 d	Amoxi/metro/pepto
56	Neg	+	14 d	Amoxi/metro/pepto
57	Neg	Neg	14 d	Amoxi/metro/pepto
58	+	Low +	14 d	Amoxi/metro/pepto
59	Neg	+	14 d	Amoxi/metro/pepto
68	Neg	Neg	14 d	Amoxi/metro/pepto
61 Household 3	+	+	14 d	Amoxi/metro/pepto
62 Household 3	+	Neg	14 d	Amoxi/metro/pepto
66 Household 4	Neg	+	7 d	Amoxi/metro/pepto
67 Household 4	Neg	Neg	7 d	Amoxi/metro/pepto

Abbreviation: PCR, polymerase chain reaction.

[a] Enroflox/metro/pepto: enrofloxacin (Baytril) 8.5 mg/kg/d divided q 12 h; metronidazole 20 mg/kg q 12 h; bismuth subsalicylate (Pepto-Bismol) 7.5 mg/kg q 12; all treatment 21 days. Amoxi/metro/pepto: amoxicillin 30 mg/kg q 12 h; metronidazole 20 mg/kg q 12 h; bismuth subsalicylate 7.5 mg/kg q 12 h; all treatment 21 days.

PCRs done by Research Associates Laboratory, R.A.L. Inc.; 14556 Midway Rd, Dallas, Texas. (Courtesy of Dr. Angela Lennox and Ernie Coliazzi.)

and tubes used to collect diagnostic material. Fig. 8 demonstrates swab insertion and gastric massage to collect the sample.

Treatment regimens

Because the ferret is used as a model for human disease, a number of treatment regimens have been devised and tested for efficacy. All involve combinations of medications, some of which need to be compounded for ease of administration to the ferret. Although *H mustelae* may be eradicated in an individual ferret, if there are other ferrets in the household, reinfection can occur. Treating the entire household of ferrets is one option, although logistically difficult for owners of multiple ferrets. Table 2 lists drug combinations used in ferrets to eradicate *H mustelae* [28,30,31]. Table 3 lists adjunctive medications for symptomatic treatment [28,30,32]. Table 4 examines effectiveness of two combination protocols as monitored by oral or gastric swab PCR posttreatment.

Treatment failures are usually linked to organism resistance to the therapeutics. As shown in Table 3, location of sample taken may alter evaluation of efficacy as well. An oral swab alone may falsely indicate clearance, although in two cases gastric swabs were negative on PCR and oral were positive. These data have not been analyzed for statistical relevance. In the trial illustrated in Table 3, the twice daily treatment using amoxicillin, metronidazole, and bismuth subsalicylate does not seem to be as effective as the use of the enrofloxacin combination. However, results may differ using different regimens, and in different populations of ferrets. Neither regimen was completely successful in eliminating the organism from all the ferrets in a particular household. In humans, resistance usually involves metronidazole, which has likely been used previously. In general, resistance to therapeutics against helicobacteriosis is increasing [28].

In summary, although *H mustelae* is found in most adult ferrets, it is not always implicated in clinical gastritis or ulcers. It does play a role as an opportunist, and exacerbates ulceration of the stomach and intestines. It appears to play a role in the development of gastric neoplasia, and may play a role in inflammatory bowel disease and colitis. As *H mustelae* is a model for human *H pylori* infection, further improvements in clinical implications, diagnosis, and treatment will be forthcoming.

We thank Dr. Angela Lennox, Ernie Coliazzi, the Washington Ferret Rescue & Shelter ferrets and volunteers, Dr. Michelle Hawkins, and the Farscape Kids.

References

[1] Evans HE, An NQ. Anatomy of the ferret. In: Fox JG, editor. Biology and diseases of the ferret. 2nd edition. Baltimore: Williams & Wilkins; 1998. p. 19–69.
[2] Staunton E, Smid SD, Dent J, et al. Triggering of transient LES relaxations in ferrets: role of sympathetic pathways and effects of baclofen. Am J Physiol 2000;279:G157–62.
[3] Blackshaw LA, Staunton E, Lehmann A, et al. Inhibition of transient LES relaxations and reflux in ferrets by GABA receptor agonists. Am J Physiol 1999;277:G867–74.
[4] Blackshaw LA, Staunton E, Dent J, et al. Mechanisms of gastro-oesophageal reflux in the ferret. Neurogastroenterol Motil 1998;10(1):49–56.
[5] Hyland NP, Abrahams TP, Fuchs K, et al. Organization and neurochemistry of vagal preganglionic neurons innervating the lower esophageal sphincter in ferrets. J Comp Neurol 2001;430(2):222–34.

[6] Smid SD, Young RL, Cooper NJ, et al. $GABA_BR$ expressed on vagal afferent neurons inhibit gastric mechanosensitivity in ferret proximal stomach. Am J Physiol 2001;281: G1494–501.

[7] Smid SD, Blackshaw LA. Vagal ganglionic and nonadrenergic noncholinergic neurotransmission to the ferret lower oesophageal sphincter. Auton Neurosci 2000;86(1–2):30–6.

[8] Abrahams TP, Partosoedarso ER, Hornby PJ. Lower oesophageal sphincter relaxation evoked by stimulation of dorsal motor nucleus of the vagus in ferrets. Neurogastroenterol Motil 2002;14(3):295–304.

[9] Page AJ, Blackshaw LA. An in vitro study of the properties of vagal afferent fibres innervating the ferret oesophagus and stomach. J Physiol 1998;512(Pt3):907–16.

[10] Rudd JA, Cheng CH, Naylor RJ. Serotonin-independent model of cisplatin-induced emesis in the ferret. Jpn J Pharmacol 1998;78(3):253–60.

[11] Van Sickle MD, Oland LD, Ho W, et al. Cannabinoids inhibit emesis through CB1 receptors in the brain of the ferret. Gastroenterology 2001;121(4):767–74.

[12] Partosoedarso ER, Abrahams TP, Scullion RT, et al. Cannabinoid1 receptor in the dorsal vagal complex modulates lower oesophageal sphincter relaxation in ferrets. J Physiol 2003; 550(1):149–58.

[13] Odekunle A, Chinnah TI. Brainstem origin of duodenal vagal preganglionic parasympathetic neurons. A WGA-HRP study in the ferret (*Mustela putorius Furo*) human model. West Indian Med J 2003;52(4):267–72.

[14] Nagakura Y, Kiso T, Miyata K, et al. The effect of the selective $5\text{-}HT_3$ receptor agonist on ferret gut motility. Life Sci 2002;71(11):1313–9.

[15] Solnick JV, Schauer DB. Emergence of diverse Helicobacter species in the pathogenesis of gastric and enterohepatic disease. Clin Microbiol Rev 2001;14(1):59–97.

[16] Fox JG, Otto G, Taylor NS, et al. *Helicobacter mustelae*-induced gastritis and elevated gastric pH in the ferret (*Mustela putorius furo*). Infect Immun 1991;59(1):1875–80.

[17] Fox JG, Paster BJ, Dewhirst FE, et al. *Helicobacter mustelae* isolation from feces of ferrets: evidence to support fecal-oral transmission of gastric Helicobacter. Infect Immun 1992;60: 606–11.

[18] Croinin TO, Clyne M, Appelmelk BJ, et al. Antigastric autoantibodies in ferrets naturally infected with *Helicobacter mustelae*. Infect Immun 2001;69(4):2708–13.

[19] Fox JG, Marini RP. Helicobacter mustelae infection in ferrets: pathogenesis, epizootiology, diagnosis, and treatment. Semin Avian Exotic Pet Med 2001;10(1):36–44.

[20] Rice LE, Stahl SJ, McLeod CG Jr. Pyloric adenocarcinoma in a ferret. J Am Vet Med Assoc 1992;200:1117–8.

[21] Erdman SE, Correa LA, Coleman MD, et al. *Helicobacter mustelae*-associated gastric MALT lymphoma in ferrets. Am J Pathol 1997;151:273–80.

[22] Garcia A, Erdman SE, Xu S, et al. Hepatobiliary inflammation, neoplasia, and argyrophilic bacteria in a ferret colony. Vet Pathol 2002;39:173–9.

[23] Saunders KE, Shen Z, Dewhirst FE, et al. Novel intestinal Helicobacter species isolated from cotton-top tamarins (*Saginus oedipus*) with chronic colitis. J Clin Microbiol 1999;37(1): 146–51.

[24] Fox JG, Rogers AB, Whary MT, et al. *Helicobacter bilis*-associated hepatitis in outbred mice. Comp Med 2004;54(5):571–7.

[25] Myles MH, Livingston RS, Franklin CL. Pathogenicity of *Helicobacter rodentium* in A/JCr and SCID mice. Comp Med 2004;54(5):549–57.

[26] Oliveira AG, das Gracas Pimenta Sanna M, Rocha GA, et al. Helicobacter species in the intestinal mucosa of patients with ulcerative colitis. J Clin Microbiol 2004;42(1):384–6.

[27] Bohr UR, Glasbrenner B, Primus A, et al. Identification of enterohepatic Helicobacter species in patients suffering from inflammatory bowel disease. J Clin Microbiol 2004;42(6): 2766–8.

[28] Lennox AM. Working up mystery anemia in ferrets. Exotic DVM 2004;6(3):22–6.

[29] Johnson-Delaney CA. A clinician's perspective on ferret diarrhea. Exotic DVM 2004;6(3): 27–8.

[30] Johnson-Delaney CA. Ferrets. In: Johnson-Delaney CA. Exotic companion medicine handbook for veterinarians. Palm Beach: ZEN Publishing; 1996. p. 1.

[31] Marini RP, Fox JG, Taylor NS, et al. Ranitidine bismuth citrate and clarithromycin, alone or in combination, for eradication of *Helicobacter mustelae* infection in ferrets. Am J Vet Res 1999;60(10):1280–6.

[32] Carpenter JW, Mashima TY, Rupiper DJ. Ferrets. In: Exotic animal formulary. 2nd edition. Philadelphia (PA): WB Saunders; 2001.

ELSEVIER
SAUNDERS

VETERINARY
CLINICS
Exotic Animal Practice

Vet Clin Exot Anim 8 (2005) 213–225

Gastrointestinal Diseases of the Ferret

Angela M. Lennox, DVM, DABVP-Avian

Avian and Exotic Animal Clinic, 9330 Waldemar Road, Indianapolis, IN 46268, USA

Gastrointestinal (GI) disease is common in pet ferrets. According to Delaney, unique ferret anatomy and physiology, including rapid GI transit time, and short, simple GI tract predisposes to GI disease [1]. Etiologies include bacteria, including helicobacter infections, virus, parasites, inflammatory conditions, neoplasia, foreign body-related diseases, and stress. Some practitioners report improvement in some refractory cases with diet modification, which suggests dietary allergen or intolerance. A thorough workup is critical for distinction between etiologies typically producing similar clinical signs and symptoms [1,2].

Diarrhea is one of the most common presenting complaints, and can represent a myriad of underlying and multifactorial causes (Fig. 1). Table 1 includes common and uncommon causes of diarrhea in pet ferrets. History can be helpful in determining underlying cause. Ferrets under 1 year of age are more prone to foreign body ingestion, coccida and proliferative colitis, while coronavirus and *Helicobacter mustelae* typically affect older ferrets [1,2].

Diarrhea occurring soon after introduction of a new ferret into the household suggests an infectious etiology, such as coronavirus, coccidia, or possibly giardia. Infectious agents such as *Lawsonia* and *Mycobacteria*, however, tend to affect only a few members of a group [1,2].

Common causes of gastrointestinal disease in ferrets

Foreign body ingestion

Ingestion of foreign material, in particular objects made of rubber or rubber-like materials, is common in ferrets under 2 years of age. Symptoms vary depending on volume of material ingested and presence of complete or partial blockage. The most common symptoms are sudden onset of

E-mail address: BirdDr@aol.com

LENNOX

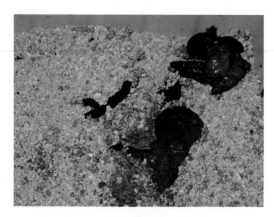

Fig. 1. Various forms of diarrhea in the ferret.

anorexia, vomiting, nausea, and lethargy, which is sometimes accompanied by stress-related diarrhea. Palpation often reveals gastric distention, GI pain, or in many cases, presence of the foreign material itself. Laboratory analysis is nonspecific, but may reflect dehydration, stress, and starvation in chronic cases. Plain radiography often reveals characteristic GI gas patterns typical of obstruction in other small animals. In some cases, definitive diagnosis is made at exploratory surgery [2].

It should be noted that the author has discovered foreign material within the stomach of ferrets undergoing abdominal surgery for reasons unrelated to GI disease. Therefore, any exploratory surgery in a ferret should include careful examination and palpation of the stomach and intestinal tract, and collection of appropriate biopsy samples.

Bacterial diseases

Ferrets are prone to both primary and secondary bacterial infections. Secondary bacterial overgrowth is not uncommon in ferrets with other diseases affecting the GI tract. Ferrets can be exposed to *Salmonella* and *Campylobacter* from ingestion of raw meat. *Escherichia coli* has been cultured from the feces of ferrets with diarrhea [2].

H mustelae is a common inhabitant of the ferret stomach, and some authors suggest prevalence in pet ferrets to be 100%. *Helicobacter* apparently does not cause disease in all ferrets, but is linked to severe lymphocytic plasmacytic inflammatory gastric lesions, diarrhea, anemia, and chronic wasting. Diarrhea can be black and tarry when *Helicobacter*-associated ulceration is present (Fig. 2). *Helicobacter* can be difficult to completely eradicate. As reinfection is common, the organism must be eliminated from all contact animals as well [3,4]. Gastric biopsies of ferrets that have undergone *Helicobacter* treatment can reveal healing ulcers, fibrosis, and other evidence of gastric damage that may explain why

Table 1
Diseases producing intermittent or chronic diarrhea in ferrets

Disease	Diagnosis	Treatment
Bacterial, primary or secondary *Helicobacter* *Lawsoni/Desulfovibrio* *Campylobacter jejuni*	Culture and sensitivity *Helicobacter* PCR, histopathology Biopsy and histopathology Culture difficult	Appropriate antimicrobial therapy, preferably based on culture and sensitivity
Bacterial, uncommon Mycobacteriosis	Histopathology PCR	Appropriate antimicrobial therapy; treatment for mycobacteriosis is controversial due to potential zoonosis
Viral; Ferret Enteric coronavirus (FEVC) Rotavirus canine distemper virus	Coronavirus isolation PCR PCR PCR	Supportive care
Coccidiosis Giardiasis	Fecal floatation, direct smear	Anticoccidial drugs
Helicobacter mustelae	PCR—gastric swab Histopathology—gastric	Specific *Helicobacter* therapy, usually triple drug therapy; traditional therapy includes metronidazole, amoxicillin and bismuth subsalicylate; other drugs including proton-pump inhibitors have been utilized
"Inflammatory bowel disease"	Histopathology	Some suggest anti-inflammatory drugs; caution in ferrets with possible *Helicobacter* or underlying bacterial or viral disease
Gastrointestinal neoplasia	Histopathology	Surgical excision Chemotherapy
Foreign body ingestion	PE, radiographs, exploratory surgery	Surgery
Stress—medical or psychologic	History Detection of underlying medical condition	Correction of underlying medical disorder or psychological stress
Idiopathic megaesophagus	Radiology	Unrewarding

treatment of *Helicobacter* does not always result in complete resolution of clinical signs (D. Reavill and R. Schmidt, personal communication, Zoo and Exotic Pathology Service, West Sacramento, CA).

Recent work in humans and laboratory animal models indicates that *Helicobacter* is not confined to the stomach and duodenum, and may play a role in inflammatory disease along the entire GI tract. In mice,

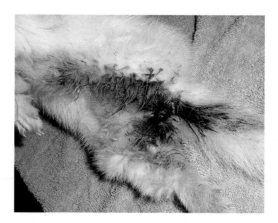

Fig. 2. Melena in a ferret with confirmed gastric ulceration.

inflammatory bowel disease is directly linked to the presence of certain subspecies of *Helicobacter*. It is currently unknown whether this link exists in the ferret, but must be considered [5–7].

Proliferative bowel disease is thought to be caused by an organism similar to that causing proliferative ileitis of pigs and hamsters. Older literature refers to the causative agent as a *Campylobacter*-like organism [2]. However, experimental infection with *Campylobacter jejunum* failed to produce lesions of proliferative bowel disease [8]. The organism was later tentatively identified as *Lawsonia intracellularis*. However, a more recent study showed that lesions typical of proliferative bowel disease could be produced by coinfection of ferrets with an intracellular *Desulfovirbio* species and coccidia [9]. Typical symptoms include chronic diarrhea with or without blood or mucus, tenesmus, and possible rectal prolapse. Weight loss and dehydration typically follow [2].

Campylobacter jejuni does occasionally cause diarrhea in ferrets younger than 6 months of age. It is usually self-limiting, and experimental studies show the disease to typically be asymptomatic. A more serious concern, however, is the potential zoonotic risk of *Campylobacter* species [2].

Mycobacteria have been isolated from the GI tract of ferrets, including granulomatous enteritis caused by *M avium,* and a disseminated gastric lesion produced by *M celatum* (type 3). Granulomatous enteritis can produce vomiting, anorexia, and diarrhea in the affected ferret [10,11].

Diagnosis of bacterial diseases is often not straightforward (Table 2). Many of the organisms mentioned above are not readily identified using standard culture and sensitivity methods.

Viral diseases

Viruses producing GI disease in ferrets include coronavirus, rotavirus, and canine distemper virus [12]. It should be kept in mind that any viral disease that does not primarily affect the GI tract may produce diarrhea secondary to stress and general debilitation.

Rotavirus has been documented in several large ferret facilities worldwide, and typically affects animals 4 to 6 weeks of age. Morbidity is high in this age group, and low in adult ferrets. Younger ferrets may die of secondary complications including dehydration. Rotavirus does not appear to be a commonly diagnosed disease of ferrets in the pet population but must be considered a potential diagnosis in very young animals [2]. Polymerase chain reaction (PCR) testing is currently available to detect Rotavirus in suspect ferrets (M. Kuipel and R. Maes, personal communication, Michigan State University, Department of Pathobiology and Diagnostic Investigation; kiupel@dcpah.musu.edu).

Canine distemper virus can produce diarrhea in affected ferrets, along with more typical symptoms including ocular and nasal discharge, characteristic skin rash, and so-called "hard pad" [2]. PCR, immunohistochemistry, and fluorescent antibody staining, as well as virus isolation are commercially available for the postmortem diagnosis of canine distemper virus (M. Kuipel and R. Maes, personal communication, Michigan State University, Department of Pathobiology and Diagnostic Investigation; kiupel@dcpah.musu. edu) [13]. PCR product can also be sequenced to differentiate field strains from vaccine strains [13]. Canine distemper virus can also be identified through immunohistochemistry of ante-mortem intestinal biopsy specimens.

Table 2
Diagnosis of bacteria producing gastrointestinal diseases in ferrets

Bacterial organism	Definitive diagnosis
Salmonella sp, E coli, Enterobacter sp, other	Standard aerobic culture and sensitivity; consider anaerobic culture as well
Helicobacter mustelae	Culture difficult
	Polymerase chain reaction (PCR) gastric mucosal, colonic, and mouth swabs
	Histopathology of gastric samples
Lawsonia intracellularis (Desulfovibrio spp)	Histopathology of colonic biopsy samples
Campylobacter jejuni	Special culture and sensitivity requirements; contact diagnostic laboratory
	Dark-field microscopy of fresh feces to observe motility characteristics of organism
Mycobacterium spp	Biopsy of gastrointestinal lesions
	Acid-fast staining of suspected lesions
	PCR of suspected lesions

Data from Lennox AM. Working up mystery anemia in ferrets. Exotic DVM 2004;6(3):22–6; and Williams BH. Ferret microbiology and virology. In: Fudge A, editor. Laboratory medicine, avian and exotic pets. Philadelphia: WB Saunders; 2000.

In 1993, breeders and veterinarians recognized an outbreak of diarrhea later termed epizootic catarrhal enteritis (ECE). Typical presentation included profuse green diarrhea with excessive mucus. Although morbidity was typically high, mortality was generally low with supportive care. Older ferrets with a concurrent disease were often most severely affected. Typical history included an onset of diarrhea in existing pets shortly after introduction of new, apparently normal, ferrets into the household. Incubation period is typically 48 to 72 hours. Older ferrets that recover from ECE often developed chronic diarrhea and wasting [14].

Coronavirus particles were identified by transmission electron micros-copy in feces and jejunal specimens, and by immunohistochemical staining of jejunal sections. Histopathologic lesions of intestine also were typical of coronaviral infection [14]. Recent work has now classified the virus as a novel ferret coronavirus, and suggested the name ferret enteric coro-navirus (FECV). PCR testing is now commercially available, and has been shown to reliably identify FECV in the feces, saliva, and intestinal biopsy specimens of infected ferrets [15].

Inflammatory gastrointestinal disease

By definition, inflammatory GI disease is the accumulation of in-flammatory cells within samples of the GI system or organs. Classification largely depends on the types and proportions of cells identified, and location of the inflammatory process. Some pathologists classify lymphocytic/plasmacytic inflammation of the intestine as "inflammatory bowel disease." The presence of moderate to large numbers of eosinophils may warrant a histologic diagnosis of "eosinophilic gastroenteritis" [2]. It is uncertain whether or not specific etiologies produce specific patterns of inflammatory infiltrate allowing definitive diagnosis. Several authors believe eosinophilic inflammatory infiltrate to be more indicative of an allergic response, perhaps to dietary antigen [2,5]. Much work remains to be done on the etiology and pathogenesis of inflammatory GI disease in ferrets.

Of 135 cases of ferret GI organ and lymph node biopsies submitted to an exotic animal pathology laboratory, 92% reported mild to severe in-flammation (Zoo and Exotic Pathology Service, Drs. Reavill and Schmidt, personal communication). Of these submissions, 73% reported symptoms related primarily to the GI tract, such as vomiting and diarrhea. The rest reported less specific symptoms such as weight loss and anorexia, or no symptoms recognized at all. In the latter cases, samples were most often collected during exploratory surgery to investigate adrenal disease, or other non-GI indication. Severity of the lesion did not always correlate with severity of clinical symptoms. Spiral organisms consistent with *Helicobacter* sp. were identified in gastric samples with varying types and severities of inflammatory infiltration [5]. It has been speculated by Johnson-Delaney that ferrets may have aberrations with one or more tumor suppressor genes.

The ferret's response to infection with Helicobacter may be further explained through examination of the genome and enteric immune responses. Research is currently underway to explore this possibility.

Neoplasia

GI neoplasia commonly presents as vague GI symptoms. The author has seen disseminated intestinal lymphoma on several occasions, and symptoms have ranged from acute death due to intestinal perforation without previous symptoms, to chronic or intermittent diarrhea (Fig. 3).

GI neoplasia has been linked to *Helicobacter* sp. infections in both humans and ferrets, and includes lymphoma, adenocarcinoma, and recently colonic adenomas in humans [3,4,16]. Recent cases of pyloric adenocarcinoma in ferrets presented as intermittent vomiting, and most advanced cases have palpably enlarged stomachs [17,18]. A case of adenocarcinoma of the colon presented as rectal prolapse [5].

Changes suggesting lymphoid neoplasia are commonly reported in enlarged gastric and mesenteric lymph nodes submitted for histopathology. In some cases differentiation of reactive versus neoplastic lymph nodes is difficult.

Miscellaneous

Megaesophagus has been diagnosed in ferrets. Clinical signs include difficulty swallowing, decreased appetite, and regurgitation. Treatment included fluids, antibiotics and agents directed against possible primary causes of megaesophagus, and were reported as ineffective. Nine ferrets ultimately submitted for necropsy and histopathology had no etiology determined for megaesophagus [19].

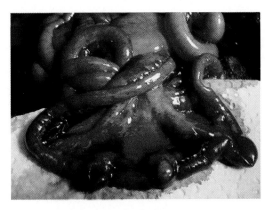

Fig. 3. Intestinal lymphoma and bowel perforation. This ferret had experienced mild intermittent diarrhea for several weeks before presenting with acute depression and anorexia.

Cryptococcus has been reported in the literature as a cause of GI disease in a ferret. The organism was identified in a section of intestine of a ferret that exhibited vague GI symptoms [20].

Diagnosis of gastrointestinal disease

Clinical pathology

Complete blood count (CBC) and chemistry panel can provide clues to diagnosis and help evaluate overall patient condition. In many cases biochemical changes simply reflect patient dehydration, anorexia, and wasting. Anemia can occur from chronic inflammation and blood loss Table 3 lists typical complete blood count and biochemistry testing changes expected with typical GI diseases of ferrets [21].

Culture and sensitivity can help identify primary or secondary bacterial pathogens. *H mustelae* is a common pathogen of ferrets, but cannot be identified on culture. Biopsy and histopathology of gastric samples, or PCR of gastric, colonic, or mouth swabs provide more specific diagnosis. As *H mustelae* is thought to be present in nearly all ferrets, and does not always produce disease, the most useful application of PCR is to monitor response to therapy and detect reinfection after successful therapy [4].

Radiography

Radiography is useful in the diagnosis of GI disease. Abnormal gas patterns can suggest foreign body obstruction or enteritis.

Contrast media have been used to evaluate the GI tract. A recent study on results of the use of barium sulfate, 8 to 13 mL/kg, indicated that small intestinal transit time was less than 2 hours. Visualization of the barium-filled small bowel was optimal at 20 and 40 minutes postbarium administration. Small bowel loops in these normal ferrets did not exceed 5 to 7 mm in width. The use of ketamine and diazepam to facilitate radiography did not significantly slow GI transit time in these ferrets [22].

Ultrasound

Abdominal ultrasonography can be an extremely effective diagnostic tool for evaluation of abdominal organs in dogs, cats, and other mammals. Information on organ size, shape, density, and even GI motility can be beneficial. The most common reported usage in the pet ferret is for evaluation of adrenal glands in ferrets with suspected adrenal neoplasia, but GI ultrasound should provide similar benefits to those reported in canine and feline practice.

Table 3
Ferret gastrointestinal diseases and common clinical pathologic changes

Disease	Clinical pathology change
Bacterial or viral enteritis	Changes depend on chronicity of disease: also commonly see elevated ALP, AST, and ALT. Changes can also reflect anorexia, starvation, and dehydration.
Gastric and/or intestinal foreign body	Changes typically reflect anorexia, starvation, stress, and dehydration: leukocytosis, neutrophilia, lymphocytosis. Elevated hematocrit and BUN may reflect dehydration
Gastritis	Same as above
Gastric ulceration	Same as above: anemia is common, positive occult fecal blood test
Proliferative bowel disease	Changes depend on chronicity of disease but often reflect dehydration, possible anemia, and hypoalbuminemia
Eosinophilic gastroenteritis	Can see marked eosinophilia, as high as 35%. Changes can also reflect anorexia, starvation, and dehydration
Megaesophagus	Changes reflect anorexia, starvation, and dehydration, depending on chronicity of disease.

Abbreviations: ALP, alkaline phosphatase; ALT, alanine aminotransferase; AST, aspartate aminotransferase.

Modified from Jenkins JR. Rabbit and ferret liver and gastrointestinal testing. In: Fudge A, editor. Laboratory medicine, avian and exotic pets. Philadelphia: WB Saunders; 2000; with permission.

Endoscopy

Rigid or flexible endoscopy can aid diagnosis of GI disease in dogs and cats. Few reports exist documenting its usefulness in ferrets, but can be expected to provide similar benefits. The author has reported use of a semiflexible 1.2-mm endoscope with air insufflation to document gastric ulceration in a ferret [4].

Laparoscopy has been described in the ferret. The technique is relatively simple, but primary use is for visualization and biopsy of those organs available for collection via simple clamshell or punch-style biopsy forceps or True-cut needles, such as liver, pancreas, and kidney [23]. Full-thickness GI biopsies in the ferret must be obtained via traditional laparotomy.

Gastrointestinal biopsy

Biopsy of GI tract remains the most specific test for confirmation of etiology, especially in those cases refractory to treatment. Diagnosis of

GI neoplasia, inflammatory GI disease, and disease secondary to unusual forms of bacteria is extremely difficult without biopsy. Biopsy and histopathology are extremely useful for monitoring response to treatment. ECE virus and canine distemper virus can also be detected in biopsy samples of the small intestine through immunohistochemistry [12,13].

In human medicine, GI biopsy remains the gold standard for diagnosis of Helicobacter-related gastroenteritis, as simple presence of the organism does not always correlate well with disease [24].

Gastric or colonic mucosal biopsy samples can be collected via semi-flexible or flexible endoscopy. Surgical biopsy during laparotomy, however, gives the added advantage of allowing visualization and targeting of grossly abnormal sections, and collection of full-thickness samples.

Miscellaneous testing

Some GI diseases such as Helicobacter-related gastric ulceration produce hematochezia. Fecal occult blood testing can help confirm the presence of blood. As some diseases produce only intermittent bleeding, a single negative occult fecal blood test does not rule out GI hemorrhage [3,4].

The Hemoccult Fecal Occult Blood Test (Beckman Coulter, www.coulter.com) has been evaluated in clinical practice for use in ferrets. Elimination of dietary heme must precede testing, and can be accomplished by feeding a nonheme-containing diet. Johnson-Delaney and Lennox demonstrated success with the use of two carnivore critical care diets (Quantum Series Enteral Carnivore Diet, Walkabout Farms, Pembroke, Virginia, www.herpnutrition.com; Oxbow Pet Products, Murdock, Nebraska, www.oxbowhay.com) [1,4].

Treatment of gastrointestinal disease

Treatment of GI disease is ideally based upon a thorough workup and a confirmed diagnosis, or at least a tentative diagnosis based on physical exam findings, and laboratory analysis. It should be noted that treatments suggested for one GI disease might exacerbate another condition. For example, drugs suggested for inflammatory bowel disease may be contraindicated when active viral or bacterial agents are present. Table 4 lists drugs commonly used to treat GI disease in ferrets.

Supportive care includes replacing fluid needs, and ensuring adequate nutrition to prevent weight loss and loss of muscle mass that often accompanies chronic diarrhea. A number of hand-feeding products have been suggested, including high-protein commercial foods such as Oxbow

Table 4
Formulary of drugs used to treat gastrointestinal disease in ferrets

Drug and dosage	Indication	Comments
Amoxicillin: 20 mg/kg bid × 28 days	*Helicobacter* "triple therapy"	Clinical trials on ferrets proven effective
Metronidazole: 30 mg/kg bid × 28 days		
Pepto Bismal: 15 mg/kg bid × 28 days		
Loperamide hydrochloride 0.2 mg/kg q12h	Supportive care	Often ineffective
Azathioprine: 0.9 mg/kg po q72h[a]	Inflammatory bowel disease	Immune suppressor; contraindicated in cases of infectious disease; monitor CBC/Chem during therapy
Enrofloxacin 5–10 mg/kg po bid	Susceptible microorganisms	
Sulfadimethoxine 50 mg/kg po, then 25 mg/kg q24h × 9 days	Coccidia	
Amprolium 19 mg/kg po q24h	Coccidia	
Metronidazole 15–20 mg/ kg po q12h × 14 days	Gastrointestinal protozoa	
Metoclopramide 0.2–1.0 mg/kg q6–8h po, sq, im	Antiemetic, motility enhancer	
Cimetidine 5–10 mg/kg po sq im q8h	H2 blocker; inhibits acid secretion; GI ulcers	Give iv slowly
Famotidine 0.25–0.50 mg/ kg po iv q24h	Inhibits acid secretion; GI ulcers	
Sucralfate 25 mg/kg po q8h	Gastrointestinal ulcers	

[a] *Data from* Burgess M, Garner M. Clinical aspects of inflammatory bowel disease in ferrets. Exotic DVM 2002;4(2):29–33.
Modified from Carpenter JW, Mishima TY, et al. Exotic animal formulary. 2nd edition. Philadelphia: WB Saunders; 2001; with permission.

Carnivore Critical Care (Oxbow Pet Products, Murdock, Nebraska, www.oxbowhay.com), Hill's a/d, strained turkey, or chicken baby food.

Antidiarrheal drugs such as loperamide hydrocloride are sometimes helpful in slowing diarrhea as an adjunct to treatment of the primary underlying cause [25].

A number of protocols have been suggested for treatment of neoplasia in ferrets, in particular GI lymphoma [25,26]. It should be noted that in humans, there is strong evidence that treatment to eradicate *Helicobacter pylori* alone may cure low-grade gastric lymphoma [27]. Therefore, clinicians treating GI neoplasia, especially those tentatively linked with *Helicobacter* sp., should consider therapy targeting at this organism as well.

GI disease is a common clinical manifestation in pet ferrets. Numerous disease conditions can produce primary GI disease, or secondary disease due to debilitation and stress. A careful and thorough workup is necessary to determine etiology and to help develop an optimal therapeutic plan.

References

[1] Johnson-Delaney CA. A clinician's perspective on ferret diarrhea. Exotic DVM 2004;6(3): 27–8.

[2] Hoefer H, Bell J. Gastrointestinal diseases. In: Quesenberry K, Carpenter J, editors. Ferrets, rabbits and rodents, clinical medicine and surgery. 2nd edition. St. Louis (MO): Saunders.

[3] Fox JG, Marini RP. *Helicobacter mustelae* infection in ferrets: pathogenesis, epizootiology, diagnosis and treatment. Sem Avian Exotic Pet Med 2001;10:36–42.

[4] Lennox AM. Working up mystery anemia in ferrets. Exotic DVM 2004;6(3):22–6.

[5] Cardonna L, Armati L. Enteric bacteria, lipopolysaccharides and related cytokines in inflammatory bowel disease: biological and clinical significance. J Endotoxin Res 2000;6(3): 205–14.

[6] Franklin CL, Riley LK, Livingston RS, et al. Enteric lesions in SCID mice infected with "Helicobacter typlonicus," a novel urease-negative Helicobacter species. Lab Anim Sci 1999; 49(5):496–505.

[7] Saunders KE, Shen Z. Novel intestinal Helicobacter species isolated from cotton-top tamarins (*Saguinus oedipus*) with chronic colitis. J Clin Microbiol 1999;37(1):146–51.

[8] Bell JA, Manning D. Evaluation of *Campylobacter jejuni* colonization of the domestic ferret intestine as a model of proliferative colitis. Am J Vet Res 1991;52(6):826.

[9] Li X, Pang J, Fox JG. Coinfection with intracellular *Desulfovibrio* species and coccidia in ferrets with proliferative bowel disease. Lab Anim Sci 1996;16(5):569–71.

[10] Valheim M, Djonne B, Heiene R, et al. Disseminated *Mycobacterium celatum* (type 3) infection in a domestic ferret (*Mustela putorius furo*). Vet Pathol 2001;38(4):460–3.

[11] Schultheiss PC, Dolginow SZ. Granulomatous enteritis caused by *Mycobacterium avium* in a ferret. J Am Vet Med Assoc 1994;204(8):1217–8.

[12] Williams BH. Ferret microbiology and virology. In: Fudge A, editor. Laboratory medicine, avian and exotic pets. Philadelphia: WB Saunders; 2000.

[13] Ramos-Vara JA, Kiupel M, et al. Diagnostic immunohistochemistry of infectious diseases in dogs and cats. J Histotech 2002;25:201–14.

[14] Williams B, Kiupel M, West KH, et al. Coronavirus-associated epizootic catarrhal enteritis in ferrets. JAVMA 2000;217(4):526–30.

[15] Wise A, Kieupel M, et al. Development and evaluation of molecular techniques for the diagnosis of epizootic catarrhal enteritis infection of ferrets. Verh Ver Erkrg Zootiere 2003; 41:427–32.

[16] Breuer-Katschinshi B, Nemes K, Marr A, et al. *Helicobacter pylori* and the risk of colonic adenomas. Colorectal Adenoma Study Group. Digestion 1999;60(3):210–5.

[17] Rice LE, Stahl SJ, McLeod CG Jr. Pyloric adenocarcinoma in a ferret. J Am Vet Med Assoc 1992;200(8):1117–8.

[18] Sleeman V, Clyde VL, Jones MP, et al. Two cases of pyloric adenocarcinoma in the ferret (*Mustela putorius furo*). Vet Rec 1995;127(11):272–3.

[19] Blanco MC, Fox JG, Rosenthal K, et al. Megaesophagus in nine ferrets. J Am Vet Med Assoc 1994;205(3):444–7.

[20] Malik R, Alderton B, Finlaison D, et al. Cryptococcosis in ferrets: a diverse spectrum of clinical disease. Aust Vet J 2002;80(12):749–55.

[21] Jenkins JR. Rabbit and ferret liver and gastrointestinal testing. In: Fudge A, editor. Laboratory medicine, avian and exotic pets. Philadelphia: WB Saunders; 2000.

[22] Schwarz LA, Solano M, Manning A, et al. The normal upper gastrointestinal examination in the ferret. Vet Radiol Ultrasound 2003;44(2):165–72.

[23] Murray MJ. Laparoscopy in the domestic ferret. Proc Int Conf Exot 2002;4:3.

[24] Munson L. Emerging helicobacter diseases. Proc Am Assoc Zoo Vet 1996;490.

[25] Carpenter JW, Mishima TY, et al. Exotic animal formulary. 2nd edition. Philadelphia: WB Saunders; 2001.

[26] Fisher P, Lennox A. Therapeutic options for ferret lymphoma: a review. J Exot Mam Med Surg 2003;1:2.

[27] Medscape Reuters Health Information. *Helicobacter pylori* eradication may cure low-grade gastric lymphoma. Gut 2004;53:34–7(www.medscape.com/viewarticle/466949).

ELSEVIER
SAUNDERS

VETERINARY
CLINICS
Exotic Animal Practice

Vet Clin Exot Anim 8 (2005) 227–245

Amphibian Gastroenterology

Leigh Ann Clayton, DVM

National Aquarium in Baltimore, Pier 3, 501 East Pratt Street,
Baltimore, MD 21202-3194, USA

The class Amphibia includes three orders with more than 4000 species. The order Anura, or Salienta, includes the frogs and toads; Caudata, or Urodela, includes the salamanders, newts, and sirens; and Gymnophiona, or Apoda, includes the caecilians [1]. This article focuses on adult anurans and urodeles because species in these orders are presented most commonly to veterinarians. A general review of caecilian medicine is available for interested readers [2]. This article begins with a discussion of larval (tadpole) and adult anatomy and physiology, because this topic is represented poorly in the veterinary literature. Common presenting signs and diagnostic techniques are reviewed, followed by a discussion of specific diseases and treatment options.

Anatomy and physiology

Larvae

Larval anurans (tadpoles) are aquatic and typically omnivorous, although species differences in feeding patterns exist [3,4]. In general, tadpoles feed by filtering particles out of the water. Water is brought actively into the mouth and directed through mucus-covered filter plates in the pharynx, which are located cranial to the gills. This filtering structure, termed the branchial sieve, has been described in detail [3]. Although the filters are fine enough to remove plankton, bacteria, and protozoa, most species seem to feed actively on larger material in the aquatic environment [3].

The lips are composed of a keratin beak [5]. A soft oral disc, covered with keratin denticles, surrounds the mouth. The denticles are used to "graze" on vegetation or animal remains; the surface is rasped to loosen organic material, which is filtered by the branchial sieve. The beak also may be used

E-mail address: lclayton@aqua.org

1094-9194/05/$ - see front matter. Published by Elsevier Inc.
doi:10.1016/j.cvex.2004.12.001

to remove larger pieces of food [5]. Specific feeding needs and strategies vary with species [3]. A detailed review of larval oral anatomy is available [6].

The filtered food material is transported by cilia into the esophagus and stomach, or fore-gut, which is short and narrow [3,7]. Peristalsis does not occur. The stomach—a small dilation at the end of the esophagus—produces no enzymes and seems to function primarily for food storage [3]. Digestion occurs in the midgut, or small intestine. The tadpole small intestine is elongated, narrow, and curled extensively within the body cavity [3,5].

During metamorphosis, dramatic changes to the larval form are reflected in the intestinal tract. The stomach widens and lengthens, and extensive glandular development occurs. The long, thin midgut shortens and widens in the adult [3,5].

Larval urodeles are anatomically more similar to the adult form than larval anurans [5]. They actively hunt under water, using a snapping motion of the well-developed jaws to take appropriate-sized prey [3]. Peristalsis moves food items through the esophagus into the stomach where peptic proteolytic enzymes begin digestion [3]. The larval intestinal tract is grossly similar to the adult form, although it shortens and widens during metamorphosis [3]; however, there is significant change in the gastrointestinal cellular composition during metamorphosis [3,5,7].

Adults

The oral cavity of adult amphibians generally is wide and large. A choana is present, although the form varies among species [3,7,8]. A detailed review of the oral cavity exists for the veterinarian [8]. The lips are poorly developed compared with those of mammals and are immobile. but flexible [3,5,7,8]. The teeth assist in holding prey [3,7,9]. With few exceptions, amphibian species secrete copious amounts of mucus from buccal epithelial glands; exceptions include *Pipa, Siren,* and *Amphiuma* [3,7]. Most species also possess salivary glands, although these may be lacking in fully aquatic species [7]. Salivary and buccal gland products do not play an active role in digestion [3].

Adult amphibians are carnivorous and actively hunt and capture a wide variety of insect and vertebrate prey. Prey capture techniques vary with species, but some general trends are reported here. A detailed review is available [10]. The tongue is specialized in terrestrial species to assist in the capture of prey [3,7,8,10,11]. In many terrestrial amphibians, the tongue can be extended for considerable distances and has a sticky coating [3,5,7,8]. In anurans, the tongue generally is attached rostrally and is extended such that the ventral–caudal surface when in the mouth becomes the dorsal–rostral surface when the tongue is "flicked out" to capture prey (Fig. 1) [7,8]. Prey is trapped by a combination of mucus that is produced by the tongue, secretions from the intermaxillary gland on the roof of the mouth, and

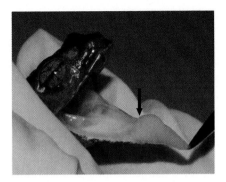

Fig. 1. Tiger-striped tree frog (*Phyllomedusa tomopterna*), postmortem. Lingual tip extended to simulate position during prey capture, note lingual attachment at rostral aspect of mandible (*arrow*).

muscular contractions of the tongue [3,5,8,10]. Species of the family Discoglossidae have lingual attachments around the entire margin of the tongue that prevent tongue extension. *Pipa* species have poorly developed tongues [3,5,10]. The tongue of terrestrial urodeles is attached along the ventral midline but can be extended out of the oral cavity when capturing prey—in some species for a distance of up to 8% of the body length [3]. Aquatic anurans and urodeles do not rely on the tongue to catch prey, and lingual development is more rudimentary [8]. They typically open their mouths quickly which creates a vacuum that pulls food and water into the oral cavity [8]. Swallowing is a coordinated movement that involves the tongue and the oral cavity [3,11]. In some anurans, retraction of the ocular globes into the oral cavity assists in moving prey into the esophagus [12].

Upper and lower esophageal sphincters are present in adult amphibians [3,7]. Esophageal contractions (peristalsis) move the food bolus into the stomach. The esophagus is lined with mucus-secreting cells and cilia that aid in this process [3,7]. Pepsinogen-secreting glands may be present within the esophagus. In some species, such as *Rana*, *Hyla,* and *Bufo*, more pepsinogen is made in the esophagus than in the stomach; however, the alkaline oral and esophageal mucus secretions prevent activation of the pepsinogen until the digesta reaches the stomach [3]. Other animals, such as *Pipa* species, produce no pepsinogen in the esophagus [3]. The esophagus of anurans is wide and short.

The esophagus and stomach are derived from the larval fore-gut, a fact that is reflected in the similarity of the secretory cells that line these organs. The histologic division between the esophagus and stomach is evident as a gradual change of cellular type and not an abrupt shift from one to the other [3,7].

The amphibian stomach lies on the left side of the body cavity. The stomach wall is composed of a glandular mucosa, thin submucosa, and well-organized tunica muscularis [3]. As in mammals, hydrochloric acid is produced in the stomach and combines with pepsinogen to form pepsins, which digest protein. The primary location for protein digestion is the stomach [7]. Under experimental conditions, the common European frog (*Rana esculenta*) had a stomach pH of 5 1 hour after ingesting an earthworm and a pH of 3 at 24 hours [3]. The effectiveness of peptic proteolysis seems to vary with temperature. Consequently, the speed of amphibian digestion is related directly to ambient temperature. The optimal temperature for digestion varies among species [3].

Muscular contractions contribute to the mechanical breakdown of the food bolus and allow mixing with digestive enzymes. Gastric contraction follows a regular pattern. A detailed summary of motility is available [3] and forms the basis of the following review. Two general types of contraction have been described in amphibians: fundic movement and pyloric movement. Fundic movement is weak but more frequent and moves soft, fluid material into the pyloric region. Pyloric movement is stronger and more dynamic but less frequent and seems to mix food materials as well as move them through the pylorus.

In experimental conditions, frogs were found to have spontaneous fundic gastric contraction at a fairly stable rate within a given temperature, although in general, contractions increased with increasing temperature. At temperatures greater than 35°C (95°F) and less than 13°C (55.4°F), contractions ceased in the bullfrog (*Rana catesbeiana*). In the mudpuppy (*Necturus* sp), spontaneous gastric contractions ceased at temperatures less than 7°C (44.6°F). In the mudpuppy, handling also can lead to cessation of gastric contractions.

Experimentally, loading the anuran stomach with food reduced the frequency of fundic contractions, whereas pyloric contractions continued. This may reflect the storage function of the fundic area, where food can be mixed with acid secretions and the pH decreased before moving into the pyloric region. Despite these local effects on spontaneous contractions, the primary control over gastric contraction seems to be effected by the midbrain or medulla [3].

The gastric brooding frog (*Rheobatrachus silus*) uses the stomach in a unique fashion. The female ingests eggs after fertilization and broods them in the fundus and proximal stomach until the young frogs are developed fully. A significant decrease in gastric acid production is achieved and is believed to be in response to a substance that is produced by the eggs, tadpoles, and young [13].

As in mammals, the amphibian stomach joins the small intestine at the gastric pyloric region. A pyloric sphincter controls release of gastric contents into the small intestine [3,7]. Most digestion occurs in the small intestine as the food bolus is mixed with secretions from the pancreas and biliary system and moved along by peristalsis. Nutrients are absorbed actively from the small intestine, as occurs in mammals [3]. In anurans, the small intestine is long and forms gentle loops within the body cavity. In urodeles, the small intestine runs directly caudally upon leaving the stomach and the looping is much reduced [3]. The small intestine of amphibians generally is simpler than in mammals, with fewer folds and villae, and is less variable along its length which makes it difficult to define specific regions (eg, duodenum, jejunum, and ileum); however, cellular composition does vary along the length of the intestine [3,7]. For instance, the cranial small intestine typically has a better developed muscular layer than more caudal sections [3].

As in mammals, the intestinal mucosa of amphibians is highly vascular and a lymphatic system is present [3,7]. Vessels that drain the intestines join the hepatic portal vein, and blood is returned to the liver. Amphibian intestines have gut-associated lymphatic tissue [14]. These aggregates of lymphoid tissue recruit lymphocytes from the circulation [14].

Typically, the liver is bilobed in anurans and undivided in urodeles. A gall bladder is present; the biliary system follows the typical mammalian pattern and function [7]. Acidic contents in the intestine stimulate release of bile from the gall bladder. Amphibian bile seems to improve digestion of fats by breaking fat particles into micelles, thus increasing the surface area upon which lipase can act [3]. A detailed review of amphibian bile composition is available [3].

The pancreas is a separate organ that is located between the duodenum and stomach in the hepato-gastric ligament. Again, structure and function in amphibians are similar to that of mammals. The number of ducts that connect the pancreas and intestine varies among species, but typically only one or two are present, although *Proteus* species may have more than 20 [3]. Amylase, lipase, and trypsin are produced by the pancreas and enter the small intestine to assist in digestion. Release of these chemicals is stimulated by secretin, which is produced in the small intestine in response to acidic ingesta [3]. Research does not support the ability of amphibian digestive enzymes to process keratin, chitin, or cellulose [3]. The pancreas also produces insulin [5].

The large intestine of amphibians generally has a greater diameter than the small intestine. In *Rana* species, a valve separates the small and large intestines. The large intestine is the primary location for water and salt absorption but is not believed to contribute significantly to digestion [3,7]. Like reptiles and birds, amphibians have a cloaca, through which the contents of the urinary, genital, and intestinal tract pass before exiting the body.

Clinical signs of gastrointestinal disease

Larvae

Larval gastroenterology is undefined in the veterinary literature, except in the broadest terms. Most gastrointestinal disease is described as part of a larger disease complex, such as bacterial sepsis or viral disease. Thus, clinical signs generally are severe and first apparent as mortalities in a group of animals. Signs of systemic disease, such as edema or cutaneous erythema, are typical; intestinal signs are not the primary complaint.

Grossly abnormal mouthparts have been found in tadpoles that were infected with chytrid fungus (*Batrachochytrium dendrobatidis*) or that have been exposed to certain toxins (such as DDT). Although the tadpoles seemed able to eat normally and showed no overt clinical signs, it is possible that such infection or exposure might influence postmetamorphosis survival [15].

Adults

As in any animal, anorexia or decreased food consumption is a general sign of illness in amphibians. Regurgitation or vomiting of food items, in this author's experience, usually is indicative of gastrointestinal disease. Gastric prolapse is a terminal sign in many species that are debilitated severely from any disease, but also can occur in response to toxins or gastrointestinal parasites [16].

Mandibular deformity (softened or shortened jaw) may occur in the early stages of metabolic bone disease [17]. Animals that hunt vigorously but are unable to capture prey may have lingual squamous metaplasia secondary to hypovitaminosis A, which decreases the "stickiness" of the tongue [18]. More commonly, inability to capture prey may be due to visual deficits that are caused by ocular or central nervous system disease.

Obstruction or impaction with food or other material may lead to obvious coelomic swelling. Overeating normal food items may result in obvious, firm gastric distention. Amphibians may present collapsed and in circulatory shock (akin to a dog that has severe gastric dilatation). Foreign object ingestion also may lead to firm, palpable masses. Other causes of palpable masses should be considered, including neoplasia or granulomas. Granulomas may caused by bacterial (typically mycobacterial), fungal, or encysted parasitic infections. In some cases, ascites is present and leads to a fluid swelling [16]. Ascites can be caused by numerous diseases, including septicemia, metabolic disease, heart failure, lymph heart failure, viral disease, or hypoproteinemia from any cause, including severe enteritis [16].

Lack of fecal production may be noted in cases of gastrointestinal impaction with food, foreign bodies, or parasites [16]. If the animal is anorexic, fecal production will be reduced; however, lack of fecal production despite a good appetite suggests early obstruction and the need for careful evaluation of the gastrointestinal tract.

Diarrhea has been associated with parasitic infection, gastroenteritis, and gastrointestinal foreign bodies [16]. Diarrhea also can be caused by feeding amphibians an inappropriate diet (eg, excess simple carbohydrates) [19]. Diarrhea must be differentiated from excess urination; however, the confirmed presence of diarrhea or mucoid stool should guide the clinician to evaluate the gastrointestinal tract.

Prolapse of the cloaca (or rectum, bladder, or oviduct) can be associated with gastrointestinal diseases, such as parasitism, foreign bodies, gastroenteritis, and neoplasias [16]. Other theorized causes of prolapse include hypocalcemia and toxins [20]. Iatrogenic cloacal prolapse can occur as a result of anesthesia with tricaine methanesulfonate (MS-222); the condition will resolve on its own during recovery [21].

Diagnostic methods

This discussion is related largely to adult amphibians, although the techniques described also can be used on larval animals. Diagnostic tests that are used in other species can be used successfully in amphibians, although modifications may be needed.

A thorough history always should be the initial diagnostic step. In amphibians, this includes a detailed review of husbandry because these species are dependent on environmental conditions to maintain basic homeostasis [22]. Key factors to investigate include temperature, humidity, light source, light cycle, substrate, cage cleaning frequency and methods, and source of water and potential water treatments. Detailed information about dietary habits must be obtained. Most amphibians are fed live invertebrate prey. If prey are not fed and cared for properly, their nutritional value will be suboptimal. In addition, detailed information about nutritional supplements should be obtained. Some species of anurans are prone to ingesting substrate with their food, which can lead to impaction. This is particularly problematic when animals are fed in naturalistic enclosures. The clinician should identify the species of animal that is being examined and be familiar with that species' basic husbandry needs.

Fecal

A fecal examination may be performed in cases of suspected gastrointestinal disease, especially if the animal is thin or has diarrhea. Direct and indirect (float) fecal examination methods should be used. Cytology also may be beneficial. The fecal analysis may reveal parasites that could be compromising the animal's health. Other abnormalities that may indicate gastrointestinal disease include an increase in undigested food, white blood cells, or budding yeast. Feces pass through the common cloaca and any material collected may, in fact, represent or include discharge from the reproductive or urinary tracts. In addition, it is helpful to collect feces from a clean container rather than the primary enclosure to minimize contamination from material in the cage.

Like most animals, amphibians may carry a variety of parasites; a detailed review of gastrointestinal parasites is available [23]. It can be difficult to determine if parasite burdens are contributing to, or are the primary cause of, clinical disease. In cases where animals are highly stressed (eg, recent shipment, improper husbandry, overcrowding), parasites can contribute to morbidity and mortality. Heavy parasite burden in an ill animal is an indication for treatment; however, low loads of potentially pathogenic organisms may not be associated with disease. Many large collections of amphibians are maintained successfully without trying to eliminate parasitic infection fully.

Amphibians carry a wide range of intestinal protozoans. The large intestine, in particular, hosts nonpathogenic protozoa [23–25]. Opalinids, for example, normally are found in the gastrointestinal flora. These rounded, multiciliated organisms exist in the colon in large numbers, are observed often in fecal examinations, and have not been associated with disease [23,25]. Coccidia infections have been reported [25].

Nematodes are present frequently in captive-bred and wild caught animals. Although generally not a concern when present in small numbers, heavy burdens can cause disease and, in severe cases, intestinal obstruction [23,25]. Pulmonary nematodes also may be present; differentiating the pulmonary and intestinal forms based on egg observation can be extremely difficult. Cestode infections have been reported and generally do not cause severe disease, although extremely heavy infections can result in intestinal obstruction [23,26]. Trematode infections have been reported in amphibians, but generally are not a significant cause of disease [25]. Encysted metacercaria can cause granulomas in any organ, including the gastrointestinal tract.

Bloodwork

Normal blood values for amphibians largely are undefined, but some preliminary references exist for a small number of species [27–29]. Blood can be obtained from many species using a variety of veins. The lingual and ventral midline veins are used commonly [21,29]. Evaluation of even a blood smear may help the clinician to appreciate changes that are associated with sepsis or neoplasia [29,30]. Protein electrophoresis may help to quantitate protein levels and identify hypoproteinemia, although detailed information on this technique is not available in the published literature [31]. Bloodwork is not the primary diagnostic test that is used in cases of gastrointestinal disease and is unlikely to provide a definite diagnosis; however, collection and evaluation always is encouraged and may provide valuable information about the patient. Generally, sedation is necessary for blood collection.

Diagnostic imaging

A detailed review of diagnostic imaging techniques for amphibians is available [32]. Techniques that are used commonly with mammals may be used with these species.

Radiographs can be helpful in delineating foreign objects (metal or stone) or confirming an obstruction. Small species will be imaged better using mammography machines or mammography film in combination with standard radiograph machines. Dental machines and film can be used for evaluating small patients if mammography equipment is unavailable.

Intestinal contrast agents (eg, barium sulfate) can be used as in mammalian medicine. In many obstruction cases, a contrast series is not required because history, clinical examination, and routine films provide adequate support for the diagnosis. Apparent hypomotility may be secondary to inappropriate environmental temperatures and stress of handling as well as general disease. Contrast agents can be delivered directly to the stomach by means of an oro-gastric tube.

Ultrasound can be used easily in amphibians. It is helpful in cases of suspected gastrointestinal disease to confirm gastrointestinal distention and poor motility. Ultrasound guidance can be used to allow fine needle aspiration of coelomic masses or fluid. Aquatic species can be imaged easily with the probe held underwater, away from the body, because ultrasound waves are conducted well through water.

CT and MRI also can be used in amphibians to help delineate masses and better define intracoelomic findings, although these techniques are not used routinely in most facilities.

Endoscopy

Coelomic or gastric endoscopy can be performed on amphibians as in other animals [16,33,34]. Rigid endoscopes or thin fiberscopes can be used to visualize the stomach and cloaca, as well as the coelomic cavity of many species. The short, wide esophagus makes gastric endoscopy easy to accomplish. The stomach can be evaluated for ulcers and foreign objects, and object removal can be accomplished with endoscopic assistance [34]. In some cases, hemostats have been used to remove gastric foreign objects that were believed to be interfering with digestion. Coelomic endoscopy may be used to visualize masses and facilitate biopsy.

Cytology/histology

Samples that are collected for cytology or histology by way of endoscopy, surgery, or necropsy can be helpful in evaluating animals that have gastrointestinal disease [33]. Submission of material from masses for evaluation by cytology or histology is the only way to differentiate their etiology. Acid-fast staining should be used routinely to evaluate all amphibian samples because mycobacterial infections are common. In some cases, however, acid-fast stains may not stain mycobacterial organisms. Non-staining rod structures should be evaluated further and a different acid-fast stain should be tried. Reliable polymerase chain reaction techniques may become readily available commercially to assist in mycobacterial diagnosis. Culture for atypical mycobacteria can be attempted but requires a laboratory that is familiar with growing these organisms. Special staining for fungal elements also should be considered in evaluating granulomas.

Full necropsies with histology, and possibly cultures, are warranted in cases of unexplained death. This is particularly important in large collections. An excellent review of the amphibian necropsy is available [35].

Common gastrointestinal diseases and treatment options

Larvae

The veterinary literature contains little information regarding identification or treatment of larval amphibian gastrointestinal diseases. Abnormal oral morphology has been related to exposure to DDT, infection with chytrid fungus, and exposure to corticosteroids [15]. Chytrid infection was reported to cause blanching of the jaw, reduction in tooth row parts, and erythema of labial papillae [15]. Toxin exposure (such as DDT) caused "cleft lip"–type abnormalities in the oral disc. Animals often are able to eat normally at this stage, and clinical signs may not be apparent without examining the mouth parts.

Viral infection with tadpole edema virus may cause gastrointestinal changes but, as the name suggests, cutaneous manifestations (eg, edema, skin hemorrhage) are more obvious [28]. Generally, this disease is diagnosed at necropsy.

Adults

Clinicians must recognize that amphibian species may vary greatly from each other, and no drug has been tested on all species. Dosages of medications mentioned in this article have been published [36]; however, readers always are encouraged to consult the literature for new information. If a clinician is faced with treating a large group of animals and is unsure if the medication may be toxic, a few animals should be tested before group treatments. Appropriate dosing in small species requires a micropipette.

Emergency case management should include: appropriate thermal support, fluid support with balanced electrolyte solutions, oxygen administration, and a clean hospital tank. Antibiotic administration should be considered pending diagnostic results because sepsis is a common finding in ill amphibians. Empiric treatment should focus on antibiotics that are effective against gram-negative organisms. The ideal fluid for general supportive care, as well as for treating specific diseases, is unknown, although some existing formulas seem to be beneficial [36].

Parasitism

Intestinal parasitism can lead to poor body condition, diarrhea, intestinal inflammation, cloacal or gastric prolapse, and physical obstruction if parasite burdens are high [28]. Although many investigators do not consider parasites to be a primary source of gastrointestinal disease in amphibians, they can exacerbate other disease processes, particularly in debilitated animals [23,28]. As usual, the clinician must interpret each case individually. If animals are highly stressed or were imported recently, treatment of identified parasites may be valuable; however, the clinician must recognize that certain parasites normally are found in the gastrointestinal tract and address any underlying husbandry factors that may be preventing the animal from mounting an adequate immune response. Complete elimination of all parasites in an individual animal or collection generally is not feasible, and may not be particularly beneficial. Treatment of potentially pathogenic parasites or of high parasite burdens is warranted, however, if these conditions are suspected factors in morbidity or mortality.

Protozoan parasites often are nonpathogenic. This is particularly true for the opalinids, and treatment should not be undertaken to reduce them. Flagellates (trichomonads, diplomands) and *Entamoeba ranarum*, however, may cause diarrhea and weight loss. Treatment with metronidazole is indicated [28].

Metazoan parasites (trematodes, nematodes, cestodes) also can cause disease, although in low numbers these parasites are seldom pathogenic. Digenea trematode cysts (metacercarial form) can form granulomas in the intestines; clinical signs generally are not apparent. Nematode infection can lead to health problems, strongylids and ascarids can cause weight loss and diarrhea, and severe infestation can lead to obstruction [28]. Infection by the cestode, *Nematotaenia*, also has been linked to weight loss and, in severe cases, obstruction [28]. *Acanthocephalus ranae* (thorny-headed worm) was reported in some amphibians and can cause enteritis and intestinal perforation. Medical treatment is considered to be ineffective [26,28]. Theoretically, surgery to remove the worms might be helpful. Coccidia parasites (eg, *Eimeria, Isospora*) also may cause diarrhea and weight loss in some animals [28].

Treatments that are used commonly in other species, such as ivermectin, fenbendazole, praziquantel, and metronidazole, can be used in amphibians [36]. Ivermectin, in particular, was reported anecdotally to cause toxicity and death in some species, although doses up to 400 µg/kg have been used without problem at this facility. Care should be taken to dose the medication appropriately in small species. In addition to possible toxicity, rapid die-off of parasites from any medication can cause severe systemic inflammatory reactions. In debilitated animals, supportive care often is warranted before treatment.

Food impaction

Certain species are prone to severe overeating, sometimes with life-threatening complications. Although the horned frogs (*Ceratophrys* spp) are particularly known for this behavior, it can occur in almost any species [19]. The resulting gastric distention can be severe enough to compromise respiratory function and induce hypovolemic shock. Emergency supportive care is essential, and prompt removal of gut contents, by way of the oral cavity or surgical gastrotomy, can be curative. If removal is by way of the oral cavity (either by gavage or directly with forceps), the clinician must take particular care; a distended stomach can be torn easily.

In other cases, distention may not be severe, but decay of food in the stomach that results from impaired digestion can result in life-threatening toxin production [19,37]. Animals also may develop impaction of the lower intestines with nondigestible portions of food items (eg, chitin insect parts). Typically, these processes are related to substandard husbandry practices that reduce digestive activity or gut motility, or contribute to dehydration. In one instance, an intestinal neoplasia caused sufficient narrowing of the intestine to prevent normal passage of nondigestible food material, which led to obstruction [38]. When disease is not the underlying factor, supportive care may be sufficient to restore normal food clearance. In other cases, surgery is needed to remove the items. Prognosis varies greatly in these cases.

Foreign object ingestion

Many amphibians have indiscriminate eating habits and can ingest significant foreign material with food items. For example, gastric bloat secondary to ingestion of plant material was reported in a wild newt (Figs. 2 and 3) [37]. Such material typically is found in the stomach or intestines, although it also can accumulate in the colon. Removal of material by way of surgery or the oral cavity generally is indicated, although in some cases, supportive care may be enough to allow the material to pass. Ideally, tank substrate should be such that it cannot be ingested when the animal feeds. Alternately, animals can be moved to a barren tank for feeding.

Prolapse

A diagnosis of cloacal prolapse is made easily during a visual examination, and the standard treatments that are used in reptiles or birds are applicable. The tissue should be kept moistened and clean, and reduction should be attempted as soon as possible. Generally, this is accomplished under sedation. As in all species, it is important to differentiate which tissue is prolapsed and identify and treat underlying diseases. Prolapse may be secondary to gastrointestinal disease, such as parasitism, foreign body, gastroenteritis, and neoplasias [28]. Prolapse also has been seen with metabolic bone disease and may be idiopathic [19,20]. Gastric prolapse through the oral cavity generally is a terminal sign,

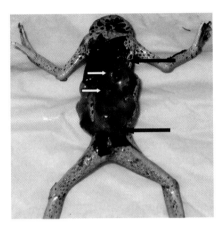

Fig. 2. Yellow and blue poison dart frog (*Dendrobates tinctorius*). Animal was found dead in cage without clinical signs; severe gastric distention from moss impaction was found at necropsy. Long black arrows delineate cranial and caudal ends of stomach. Tearing of the gastric wall is present (*white arrows*).

although it may be seen secondary to parasitic disease or toxin exposure [28].

Intussusception

Intussusception is possible, although it does not seem to be as common as prolapse, food impaction, or foreign object ingestion. Diagnosis may be difficult, but the techniques that are used in other species are applicable. Surgical correction should be attempted if the problem is identified.

Granulomatous conditions

Granulomas may be caused by several organisms. The most common etiologies are mycobacterial infections, fungal diseases (eg, chromomycosis

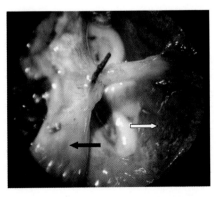

Fig. 3. Same animal as in Fig. 2. Plant material perforation of stomach with adhesion between stomach (*black arrow*) and body wall (*white arrow*). Original magnification ×10.

and mucormycosis), and encysted metazoan parasites. Inappropriate husbandry may promote the development of these conditions. Nodules may be noted in one or more locations, including the intestines, and are not always appreciated grossly. Histologic examination may be necessary to obtain a definitive diagnosis. The presence of bacterial or fungal granulomas in an amphibian warrants a detailed review of husbandry standards because suboptimal conditions can lead to a decline in the animal's immune system, with resulting development of secondary opportunistic infections [25]. In some cases, infection may represent a primary virulent pathogen [39].

Mycobacterial organisms presumably gain access by way of the cutaneous and gastrointestinal route [25,40–42]. The mycobacteria that are identified typically are environmental organisms (ie, atypical mycobacteria), such as *Mycobacterium marinum*, *M fortuitum*, and *M xenopi*. These organisms are potentially zoonotic [25]. In general, mycobacterial infections are chronic, active processes that tend to progress slowly over time [25]. Although granulomas typically are found in multiple organs, solitary lesions of the intestinal tract do occur, particularly in *Xenopus* species [25,40]. Animals may present with skin lesions or with a "wasting" syndrome, despite a good appetite.

Cytology or histology can demonstrate acid-fast, gram-positive organisms in tissue. Culture is possible and is recommended to identify the species that are involved [40]. To this author's knowledge, successful treatment of amphibian mycobacterial cases has not been reported. In general, mycobacterial infection in amphibians should be considered disseminated by the time of diagnosis.

Fungal granulomas also are reported commonly in amphibians and generally are disseminated throughout the body cavity, including the gastrointestinal tract [35,39,43,44]. Single gastrointestinal fungal granulomas are possible, although rare [26]. Fungal infection generally involves organisms that are found commonly in the environment, such as pigmented fungi of the family Dematiaceae (chromomycosis) or *Mucor* species (mucormycosis). These generally are considered to be secondary pathogens, although *Mucor amphibiorum* may behave like a primary pathogen in some species [45]. Although treatment generally is unsuccessful, one article supports the use of surgical resection and itraconazole to treat a single cutaneous nodule [46]. Theoretically, a single granuloma in the intestine could be treated similarly. To the author's knowledge, there are no reports of successful treatment of disseminated fungal granulomas.

Granulomas that result from encysted parasites generally are harmless and are diagnosed postmortem, often as incidental findings. Severe parasitism, however, compromises the intestine and leads to clinical disease, including diarrhea and signs that are consistent with hypoproteinemia (eg, coelomic effusion). Treatment options for such conditions have not been described, but supportive care with fluid therapy, feeding, and antihelmenthic therapy may be attempted.

Bacterial enteritis

Primary bacterial enteritis has not been reported in amphibians. Septicemia, however, is observed commonly and may include gastrointestinal signs, such as anorexia. Septicemia is associated frequently with cutaneous erythema, especially of the legs ("red leg" syndrome). Historically, *Aeromonas hydrophila* was believed to be the causative agent, although it is now apparent that many bacteria can cause sepsis. In most cases, sepsis is assumed to be secondary to immunosuppression from other factors, such as poor husbandry or viral infection. Healthy animals can be culture-positive for organisms that are associated commonly with septic conditions, but show no evidence of disease [28,47].

Amphibians also may carry and shed *Salmonella* [48,49], although infection seldom is associated with disease [40,49]. Because of *Salmonella*'s zoonotic potential, all amphibians should be considered as possible carriers and handled appropriately.

Viral enteritis

Viral infections are known to cause morbidity and mortality in amphibians. Descriptions are based primarily on investigations of wild populations [28]. Iridoviruses have been described in anurans and urodeles [28,50]. Diagnosis often is made postmortem. Gastrointestinal changes, such as dilated loops of bowel and hemorrhage, may be described, but are a nonspecific finding [50].

Neoplasia

Neoplasias have been reported in amphibians—more frequently in anurans than in urodeles. Gastrointestinal neoplasias generally are reported to be focal masses rather than infiltrative disease. Differentiating large masses requires cytologic or histologic methods because granulomas that are caused by bacteria (especially mycobacteria), fungal infection, or parasitic infection cannot be distinguished visually from neoplasias [35]. Acid-fast staining should be done on any mass to evaluate for mycobacterial infection. Although tumors are not reported as frequently as granulomas, neoplasia should be on the differential list. There is little published information on clinical signs that are associated with gastrointestinal neoplasia; ascites and obstruction have been reported [28].

Gastric, intestinal, and cloacal adenomas and adenocarcinomas are reported most frequently in the literature [30,38]. These tend to be focal masses, although in some cases they are metastatic. Squamous cell carcinoma of the colorectal junction also has been reported [30]. Generally, case reports are described postmortem; however, it is clear that amphibians can recover from major coelomic surgery, and resection may be a viable option. The author is unaware of any reports of chemotherapy or radiation therapy in the treatment of neoplasia in amphibians.

Nutritional disorders

"Short tongue syndrome" has been described in captive Wyoming toads (*Bufo baxteri*) [18]. Animals will attempt to capture prey but cannot bring prey items into the mouth reliably. Affected animals have squamous cell metaplasia of the lingual mucus-secreting glands, which is apparent histologically. Captive animals that had this condition had markedly decreased levels of hepatic retinol compared with nonaffected, wild animals. Lingual squamous cell metaplasia is theorized to result from hypovitaminosis A [18].

Metabolic bone disease generally is considered to be a musculoskeletal disease. Folding fractures of long bones are common, but early signs may include deformity of the mandible. As hypocalcemia occurs, gastrointestinal bloating, as well as prolapse, has been observed [19,20]. Treatment is aimed at increasing systemic calcium levels by way of medications (oral, injectable, or topical calcium administration) and the use of full-spectrum UV lights (to increase vitamin D activation and thus increase calcium absorption).

Diarrhea may be induced if amphibians are fed diets that are too high in carbohydrates, such as those that contain high levels of simple sugars from grains [19]. This is associated most often with feeding commercial foods, particularly enteral support formulas to ill frogs.

Summary

Gastrointestinal disease in amphibians commonly is due to foreign object obstruction, overconsumption of normal food items, or heavy parasite burdens. Other intestinal diseases generally show multiple systemic effects. Many diseases still are diagnosed at necropsy. Continued advances in amphibian medicine will undoubtedly lead to a better understanding of disease processes and expanded treatment options. Clinicians may use the same diagnostic and therapeutic tools that are applied to diseases in other species. Detailed references are available and interested clinicians should become familiar with them when expanding amphibian practices.

Acknowledgments

The author would like to thank Susi Ridenour Staff Librarian, A. Carter Middendorf Library, National Aquarium in Baltimore for her assistance in obtaining reference material and her enthusiasm for the project.

References

[1] Wright KM. Taxonomy of amphibians kept in captivity. In: Wright KM, Whitaker BR, editors. Amphibian medicine and captive husbandry. Malabar (FL): Krieger; 2001. p. 3–14.

[2] Mylniczenko ND. Caecilians (Gymniophona, caecilia). In: Fowler ME, Miller RE, editors. Zoo and wild animal medicine. 5th edition. St. Louis (MO): Elsevier Science; 2003. p. 40–5.

[3] Reeder WG. The digestive system. In: Moore JA, editor. Physiology of the amphibia. New York: Academic Press; 1964. p. 99–149.

[4] Wright KM. Diets for captive amphibians. In: Wright KM, Whitaker BR, editors. Amphibian medicine and captive husbandry. Malabar (FL): Krieger; 2001. p. 63–72.

[5] Zug GR. Amphibians. In: Herpetology: an introductory biology of amphibians and reptiles. San Diego (CA): Academic Press; 1993. p. 3–41.

[6] Orton GL. Larvae. In: Duellman WE, Trueb L, editors. Biology of amphibians. Baltimore (MD): Johns Hopkins University Press; 1986. p. 141–71.

[7] Olsen ID. Digestion and nutrition. In: Kluge AG, editor. Chordate structure and function. 2nd edition. New York: Macmillan; 1977. p. 270–305.

[8] Goodman G. Oral biology and conditions of amphibians. Exotic Vet Clin North Amer 2003; 6(3):467–75.

[9] Ehmcke J, Wistuba J, Clemen G. Gender-dependent dimorphic teeth in four species of Mesoamerican plethodontid salamanders (Urodela, Amphibia). Ann Anat 2004;186(3): 223–30.

[10] Noble GK. Food and feeding. In: Duellman WE, Trueb L, editors. Biology of amphibians. Baltimore (MD): Johns Hopkins University Press; 1986. p. 229–40.

[11] Wolff JB, Lee MJ, Anderson CW. Contribution of the submentalis muscle to feeding mechanics in leopard frog, Rana pipiens. J Exp Zoolog Part A Comp Exp Biol 2004;301(8): 666–73.

[12] Levine RP, Monroy JA, Brainerd EL. Contribution of eye retraction to swallowing performance in the northern leopard frog, Rana pipiens. J Exp Biol 2004;207(Pt 8):1361–8.

[13] Fanning JC, Tyler MJ, Shearman DJC. Converting a stomach to a uterus: the microscopic structure of the stomach of the gastric brooding frog Rheabatrachus silus. Gastroenterology 1982;82:62–70.

[14] Ardavin CF, Zapata A, Garrido E, et al. Ultrastructure of gut-associated lymphoid tissue (GALT) in the amphibian urodele, Pleurodeles waltlii. Cell Tissue Res 1982;224:663–71.

[15] Fellers GM, Green DE, Longcore JE. Oral chytridiomycosis in the mountain yellow-legged frog (Rana muscosa). Copeia Am Soc Ichthyol Herpetol 2001;4:945–53.

[16] Bertelsen M, Crawshaw G. 5-Minute guide to amphibian disease. ExoticDVM 2003;5(2): 23–6.

[17] Wright KM, Whitaker BR. Metabolic bone disease in amphibians. ExoticDVM 2000;1(6): 23–6.

[18] Pessier AP. "Short tongue syndrome," lingual squamous metaplasia, and suspected hypovitaminosis A in captive Wyoming toads, (Bufo baxteri). In: Proceedings of the Ninth Annual Conference of the Association of Reptilian and Amphibian Veterinarians. Reno (NV): Association of Reptilian and Amphibian Veterinarians; 2002. p. 151–3.

[19] Wright KM, Whitaker BR. Nutritional disorders. In: Wright KM, Whitaker BR, editors. Amphibian medicine and captive husbandry. Malabar (FL): Krieger; 2001. p. 73–87.

[20] Wright KM. Idiopathic disorders. In: Wright KM, Whitaker BR, editors. Amphibian medicine and captive husbandry. Malabar (FL): Krieger; 2001. p. 239–44.

[21] Lewbart SG, Stoskopf MK. Amphibian medicine: selected topics. ExoticDVM 2002;4(3): 36–9.

[22] Reichenbach-Klinke H, Elkan E. Technique of investigation. In: The principal diseases of lower vertebrates. Book II diseases of amphibians. The British Crown Colony of Hong Kong: T.F.H.; 1965. p. 209–19.

[23] Poynton SL, Whitaker BR. Protozoa and metazoan infecting amphibians. In: Wright KM, Whitaker BR, editors. Amphibian medicine and captive husbandry. Malabar (FL): Krieger; 2001. p. 193–221.

[24] Delvinquier BLJ, Freeland J. Protozoan parasites of the cane toad, Bufo marinus, in Australia. Aust J Zool 1988;36:301–16.

[25] Reichenbach-Klinke H, Elkan E. Infectious diseases. In: The principal diseases of lower vertebrates. Book II diseases of amphibians. The British Crown Colony of Hong Kong: T.F.H.; 1965. p. 220–320.

[26] Elkan E, Reichenbach-Klinke HH. Parasitic diseases. In: Color atlas of the diseases of fishes, amphibians, and reptiles. The British Crown Colony of Hong Kong: T.H.F.; 1974. p. 49–186.

[27] Cooper JE. Urodele (caudate, urodela): salamanders, sirens. In: Fowler ME, Miller RE, editors. Zoo and wild animal medicine. 5th edition. St. Louis (MO): Elsevier Science; 2003. p. 33–40.

[28] Crawshaw G. Anurans (anura, salienta): frogs, toads. In: Fowler ME, Miller RE, editors. Zoo and wild animal medicine. 5th edition. St. Louis (MO): Elsevier Science; 2003. p. 22–33.

[29] Wright KM. Amphibian hematology. In: Wright KM, Whitaker BR, editors. Amphibian medicine and captive husbandry. Malabar (FL): Krieger; 2001. p. 129–46.

[30] Stacy BA, Parker JM. Amphibian oncology. Veterinary Clin North Am Exot Anim Pract 2004;7(3):673–95.

[31] Zalais J, Cray C. Protein electrophoresis: a tool for the reptilian and amphibian practitioner. J Herpetol Med Surg 2002;12(1):30–2.

[32] Stetter MD. Diagnostic imaging of amphibians. In: Wright KM, Whitaker BR, editors. Amphibian medicine and captive husbandry. Malabar (FL): Krieger; 2001. p. 253–72.

[33] Wright KM. Surgical techniques. In: Wright KM, Whitaker BR, editors. Amphibian medicine and captive husbandry. Malabar (FL): Krieger; 2001. p. 273–83.

[34] Boggs L, Theisen S. Endoscopic removal of gastric foreign bodies in an African bullfrog, *Pyxicephalus adspersus*. Newsl Assoc Reptilian Amphib Vet 1997;7(2):7–8.

[35] Pessier AP, Pinkerton M. Practical gross necropsy of amphibians. Semin Avian Exotic Pet Med 2003;12(2):81–8.

[36] Wright KM, Whitaker BR. Pharmacotherapeutics. In: Wright KM, Whitaker BR, editors. Amphibian medicine and captive husbandry. Malabar (FL): Krieger; 2001. p. 309–30.

[37] Elkan E, Reichenbach-Klinke HH. Nutritional disorders. In: Color atlas of the diseases of fishes, amphibians, and reptiles. The British Crown Colony of Hong Kong: T.H.F; 1974. p. 195–210.

[38] Clayton LA. Clinical snapshot #1: intestinal obstruction secondary to neoplasia in a marine toad (*Bufo marinus*). Compend Contin Educ Pract Vet 2002;24(7):539,555.

[39] Berger L, Speare R, Humphrey J. Mucormycosis in a free-ranging green tree frog from Australia. J Wildl Dis 1997;33(4):903–7.

[40] Taylor SK, Green DE, Wright KM, et al. Bacterial diseases. In: Wright KM, Whitaker BR, editors. Amphibian medicine and captive husbandry. Malabar (FL): Krieger; 2001. p. 160–79.

[41] Shively JN, Songer JG, Prchal S, et al. *Mycobacterium marinum* infection in Bufonidae. J Wildl Dis 1981;17(1):3–7.

[42] Green SL, Lifland BD, Bouley DM, et al. Disease attributed to *Mycobacterium chelonae* in South African clawed frogs (*Xenopus laevis*). Comp Med 2000;50(6):675–9.

[43] Miller EA, Montali RJ, Ramsay EC, Rideout BA. Disseminated chromoblastomycosis in a colony of ornate-horned frogs (*Ceratophrys ornate*). J Zoo Wildl Med 1992;23(4):433–8.

[44] Taylor SK. Mycoses. In: Wright KM, Whitaker BR, editors. Amphibian medicine and captive husbandry. Malabar (FL): Krieger; 2001. p. 181–91.

[45] Speare R, Berger L, O'Shea P, et al. Pathology of mycomycosis of cane toads in Australia. J Wildl Dis 1997;33(1):105–11.

[46] Suedmeyer WK, Gillespie DS, Pace L. Chromomycosis in a marine toad, *Bufo marinus*. Newsl Assoc Reptilian Amphib Vet 1997;7(3):13–5.

[47] Hird DW, Diesch SL, McKinnell RG, et al. Aeromonas hydrophila in wild-caught frogs and tadpoles (*Rana pipiens*) in Minnesota. Lab Anim Sci 1981;31(2):166–9.

[48] Everard COR, Tota B, Bassett D, et al. *Salmonella* in wildlife from Trinidad and Grenada, W.I. J Wildl Dis 1979;15:213–9.

[49] Hoff GL, Hoff DM. Salmonella and Arizona. In: Hoff GL, Frye FL, Jacobson ER, editors. Diseases of amphibians and reptiles. New York: Plenum; 1984. p. 69–82.

[50] Docherty DE, Meteyer CU, Wang J, et al. Diagnostic and molecular evaluation of three iridovirus-associated salamander mortality events. J Wildl Dis 2003;39(3):556–66.

ELSEVIER
SAUNDERS

Vet Clin Exot Anim 8 (2005) 247–276

VETERINARY
CLINICS
Exotic Animal Practice

Gastroenterology for the Piscine Patient

E. Scott Weber, MSc, VMD

New England Aquarium, Central Wharf, Boston, MA 02110-3399, USA

Because fish are the largest group of vertebrates with estimates of species at 25,000 [1], piscine patients pose a great veterinary challenge for private practice, on fish farms, and in a public aquarium setting. A public aquarium may have institutional collections exhibiting greater than 500 unique species ranging from apex predator sharks and piranha, to endangered pupfish and cichlids, to venomous lionfish and stonefish, and to unique seadragon and flashlight fish species. At the New England Aquarium (NEAq), the fish collection is divided into exhibit galleries that represent different biomes, which includes a giant ocean tank, representing warm water Atlantic fish, and cold marine, temperate, tropical, and freshwater galleries with multitaxa exhibits.

The NEAq Animal Health Department treats nearly 150 cases of fish per year and oversees general quarantine for nearly another 500 to 1000 individual aquatic animals. The majority of collection fishes are clinically evaluated by the Animal Health staff similar to higher vertebrates at NEAq for both medical treatment and preventive health care. When necessary, extensive diagnostic examinations are performed on individual fish. An exception to this approach exists for large groups of schooling species, as only basic skin and gill biopsies are performed on 10% to 15% of the animals before and after quarantine to check for external evidence of disease, unless an outbreak or increased mortalities are seen in these systems. All collection and quarantine animal mortalities are necropsied for gross pathology and histology. A challenge that veterinarians face in aquarium medicine is with exhibits featuring multitaxa enclosures. Although these exhibits help create more realistic environments, they also can limit medical options, because some efficacious treatments for controlling certain fish disease outbreaks may prove fatal to the invertebrates or plants found in these displays.

In an attempt to make some sense out of fish guts, this article will break down fish gastroenterology in the following manner. First, the piscine gastrointestinal tract will be discussed anatomically: beginning with the mouth and food apprehension, through the stomach, intestines, pyloric

---

E-mail address: sweber@neaq.org

1094-9194/05/$ - see front matter © 2005 Elsevier Inc. All rights reserved.
doi:10.1016/j.cvex.2005.01.009

cecae, and with discussion on accessory organs. Basic anatomy of each gastrointestinal tract section will be complemented with some pertinent histologic considerations and some general physiologic considerations.

The second section will briefly identify some of the basic diagnostic modalities frequently used to investigate gastrointestinal disease in fish at the NEAq. This will include brief mention of ultrasound, radiography, contrast radiography, fecal testing, cloacal lavage, microbiology, endoscopy, and surgery. Many supporting topics and information on fish hematology, nutrition, neoplasia, surgery, and formularies have been written for previous Veterinary Clinics articles, and will not be greatly detailed in the context of this section [2–6].

The final section will discuss several commonly observed diseases of the gastrointestinal tract in fish. These diseases will be discussed in terms of clinical presentation, diagnosis, and treatment.

The piscine gastrointestinal tract

Because this group of vertebrates is so large, the main emphasis of this article will focus on the teleost or bony fish. This class encompasses many species most likely seen by private practitioners and housed in public aquaria. Although veterinarians in public aquaria commonly treat elasmobranchs (sharks, skates, and rays), differences in this class would warrant a separate article and greatly extend the body of this work. When possible, differences in the elasmobranchs will be noted for comparison and contrast with bony fish.

The piscine gastrointestinal tract begins with apprehension of food, which then passes through the mouth, pharynx, esophagus, stomach, intestines, and pyloric cecae, with waste elimination out the cloacae and vent. The liver and pancreas will be included with any other unique adaptations and accessory organs in fish. Also, the swimbladder will be briefly discussed, as this organ is derived from the gastrointestinal tract, although the swimbladder functions as buoyancy control for many teleosts and serves no role in digestion.

Mouth, teeth, oral pharynx, and esophagus

Anatomic considerations

Water covers 70% to 75% of the earth and provides a nearly infinite array of niches and habitats for aquatic animals. Fish, as the largest vertebrate group occupying the earth, have evolved many unique features for food apprehension in remarkably diverse aquatic environs, from coral reefs to freshwater caves to puddles, and even in terrestrial locations.

The mouth, located cranially, has several possible locations that can help discern individual species feeding habits and prey preference. The original classification of piscine mouth position from Jordan and Everman [7], in 1900, is still widely referenced today. This classification scheme has four basic mouth locations. The first position is inferior, where the mouth is ventral and somewhat caudal to the rostrum such as with many species of catfish (Ictaluridae), sturgeon (Acipenseridae), some sharks, and most rays (Rajiformes). The second classification is subterminal. In this position the mouth remains ventral but is located far rostrally. This is commonly seen with dace (*Rhinichthys*). The third position is terminal, where the mouth and jaw appear oriented ventral and cranially as seen in trout and salmon (Salmonidae), and most aquarium fish. Many of the cyprinids (goldfish, koi, and carp) seen by private practitioners have mouth positions in these second and third locations. The last position is called superior, and mouth placement is cranially and dorsally located. An aquarium species displaying an excellent example of this mouth position is the monkey fish or arawana (*Osteoglossum*).

Lips may or may not be present in fish. Associated with the mouth of many fish are appendages that serve a variety of functions. The most common types of appendages are called barbels, which serve as sensory organs for gustatory and tactile reception. These barbels are located around the mouth, nostrils, and chins of several species. An excellent example of barbels can be readily recognized on catfish species such as the channel catfish (*Ictalarus punctatus*). Some fish may have modified fins that appear near the mouth or can jut in front of the mouth. These modified fins sometimes serve as lures to attract prey near the mouth in species of fish like the monkfish (*Lophius americanus*).

Although there is a super class of fish called the agnatha, which are jawless animals, the majority of animals seen by veterinarians have bony or cartilaginous jaws similar to other vertebrates. The jaw most basically consists of a premaxilla, mandible, and maxilla, but it must be noted that the skulls and jaws of fish can be quite complicated; for more information on skull development one can refer to the three-volume text of Hankin and Hall [8]. Evans notes that the skull of fish can contain approximately 185 bones [9]. The jaws define the size and shape of the mouth or buccal cavity. This size and shape is often related to the type of prey items for a particular species. Some animals such as monkfish (*L americanus*), have large jaws that allow prey items to be eaten that may be larger than the predator itself, while other orders of fish such as sygnathids (pipefish, seahorses, and sea dragons) have small toothless tube-like mouths with fused jaws that limit prey size to brine shrimp. Fish may or may not have teeth imbedded in the jaw. Teeth can be located in several other skull bones of fish including the premaxilla, maxilla, and mandible of the jaws. In elasmobranchs, several rows of teeth may be present for continual tooth replacement, where as most teleosts replace teeth when lost. On many fish species the mouth and lips are protrusible. Teeth can also be highly specialized for individual species, ranging from incisiform-shaped teeth to fused plates for crushing mollusks and crustaceans.

After entering the mouth, the buccal or oral cavities of fish are shared by both the respiratory and digestive tract. Another anatomic feature found within the mouth or buccal cavity includes the tongue, which may be fleshy, bony, or covered with teeth. Most fish are unable to protrude the tongue. Oral valves are present inside the jaws, which help direct water flow through the gill opercula for respiration. Water and food pass through the pharynx and are directed through either the gill opercula or down the esophagus. As water is directed through the opercular flaps past gills for respiration and waste exchange, food can be trapped by specialized bones called gill rakers, and then swallowed or further processed by pharyngeal teeth before traveling to the stomach. Gill rakers are highly variable in fish and can form blunted teeth or filter baskets. Many species of herbivorous fish have dorsal and ventral pharyngeal teeth or pads, which oppose each other to further pulverize or grind plant material or prey items.

After food passes through the pharyngeal region it enters the esophagus, which in most fish is short, greatly distensible, and muscular. The esophagus consists of multiple longitudinal folds. In elasmobranchs, the surface of the esophagus is lined with caudally oriented branched papillae. In the physostomous species of fish, a small duct connects the esophagus and swimbladder to allow filling of the swimbladder with air.

Histology

Histologically, the mouth contains many sensory nerve endings used for taste. The buccal and pharyngeal cavities are stratified squamous epithelium on a thick basement membrane attached to bone or muscle by a condensed dermis [10]. Unlike in mammals, the buccal and pharyngeal regions are not distinct. Numerous goblet cells are found throughout the epithelium in these areas and vary according to species. Because of the numerous bones and teeth in many species of fish, histologic fixation can be difficult. The mucosal layer of the esophagus is largely stratified epithelium with columnar or cuboidal cells that may or may not contain cilia. The muscular mucosa of the esophagus is longitudinal striated muscle in most fish. In some rare exceptions of fish, circular smooth muscle may also be present around the striated layer or the esophagus may be only circular smooth muscle. Numerous mucous secreting goblet cells and some multicelluar glands are present along the esophagus to help lubricate food for passage into the stomach [11]. Gastric glands may occur in the caudal region of the esophagus. Although the esophagus may terminate at the cardiac sphincter or valve, in many species a clear demarcation between esophagus and stomach or intestine is not readily evident. In sharks and rays, lymphomyloid material is present in the submucosal layer of the esophagus and called the organ of Leydig.

Physiologic considerations

Unlike in mammalian vertebrates, when food enters the mouth there is little or no chemical processing. Fish do not have salivary glands capable of producing salivary amylase. Mucous-producing goblet cells in the buccal cavity and the esophagus help to lubricate food for swallowing. Fish can obtain prey by a variety of ways, and the three most commonly recognized feeding behaviors are biting, used by many sharks and predatory fish; suction feeding, associated with many algae eaters or specialized feeders such as seahorses; and ram feeding, for taking in large numbers of small prey such as whale sharks. There are variations and modifications of each of these methods for the many species of fish that exist.

Extensive feeding relationships have been studied for fish, and it is thought that niche species of feeding developed only 50 million years ago from unspecialized nocturnal carnivores that comprised most fish at the time. This radiation allowed fish to evolve diurnal behavior, and feed on benthic invertebrates, coral polyps, plankton feeders, and become more specialized carnivores [12]. Fish are commonly grouped by diet, as other vertebrates. These groups include herbivores, which ingest algae or benthic plants by either grazing as parrot fish (Scaridae), or browsing like carp (Cyprinidae). There are detritivores, which depend on nonliving organic matter scooped from sediments. Many species found in captivity are carnivores because of the ease to make and prepare commercially available foods for this group. Horn [13] further divides the carnivores into plankton feeders, benthic invertebrate feeders, and piscivorous fish.

The primary action of the mouth, jaws, teeth, pharynx, and esophagus is to apprehend, mechanically breakdown, and separate food via gill rakers from water and debris, and then swallow the food with lubrication from mucous-producing cells and glands. Chemical digestion does not take place until food enters the stomach or intestine.

Stomach and pyloric cecae

The stomach and rest of the gastrointestinal tract lies within the peritoneal cavity of fish. Stomach anatomy in fish is highly variable, ranging from a barely discernable enlarging of the esophagus in sea horses to a thick-walled gizzard-like organ in certain surgeonfish (Acanthuridae). The stomach is often absent in most larval fish and in about 10% to 15% of adult species. The stomach in many species of teleosts and elasmobranchs is sigmoidal or J-shaped, but there are tremendous other teleost variations. It is highly distensible in most species of fish, and posses significant folds that form multiple rugae. Fish such as monkfish (*L americanus*), can ingest greater than 50% of their body weight at a single feeding, while other fish, like tetras (Characidae), have smaller stomach capacities that hold roughly 10% of body weight [12]. As in other vertebrate animals, the fish stomach has a cardiac and pyloric region. The stomach in many species has muscular and gastric components, although species that are agastric are not uncommon. In some herbivorous animals the stomach is round and very thick walled. In several species of fish, blind-ended pouches or diverticula, numbering a couple to over a thousand, called pyloric cecae, are found at the pyloric opening to the duodenum and are used for food absorption.

Histology

The gastric mucosa consists of a stratum compactum with fibroelastic cells and a muscularis of smooth muscle. Goblet cells are scattered throughout the stomach epithelium. Striated muscle entering from the esophagus may extend into the stomach's cardiac region, but changes to circular muscle. The layers of the muscular stomach consist of inner circular muscle surrounded by longitudinal muscle layers of smooth muscle, connective tissue, and eosinophilic granular cells. The gastric portion of the stomach is marked by an increase in numerous glands at the base of the folds resembling chief cells in other vertebrates, and some gastric glands also contain tubules similar to oxyntic cells found in higher vertebrates, which contain zymogen-like secretory granules that are released by exocytosis [12]. Pyloric cecae share a similar histologic composition with the intestine rather than the stomach. Gizzard-like stomachs generally have a cuticle-like lumen lining with several layers of smooth muscle. In animals that contain a pyloric sphincter, a thickened area of circular smooth muscle is present at this opening.

Physiologic considerations

The stomach is a site of further mechanical breakdown, and marks the beginning of chemical digestion in fish. In species such as surgeonfish (Acanthuridae) and others that possess a gizzard-like stomach, the majority of digestion is still mechanical. The presence of sand in the gizzard helps triturate algae ingested by these species. Chemical digestion occurs in the stomach for several fish species. Some fish depend on acid production to create a low pH environment similar to other vertebrates to activate enzymatic cascades for food breakdown. Gastric glands in the stomach produce pepsin, but other enzymes produced in the stomach have also been described [13]. Pepsin and low pH are primarily responsible for the chemical digestion of food at this point of digestion. Digestion and absorption in the pyloric cecae is similar to the intestine.

Intestines, anus, and cloaca

Anatomic considerations

The length of the intestine varies in fish, similar to higher vertebrates with carnivorous animals having short tracts and herbivorous fish having long intestinal tracts. Herbivorous fish often have an elongated gastrointestinal system that may be several times (up to 20 times) the length of the animal's body, with coiled intestines like in koi (*Cyprinus carpio*). Carnivorous fish often have a very short digestive tract (one fifth of the body length), often only as long as the distance between the mouth and anus as seen in trout (Salmonidae) [12]. Fish exhibit every permutation of gut length in between these extremes.

In most fish, the small and large intestine are not distinguishable grossly, although functional distinctions in different areas of the bowel seem to be present in several fish species. Most elasmobranchs have bowel segments that are observably different, and the most noticeable difference is the presence of an enlarged spiral shaped colon or valve segment (Fig. 1). The intestines terminate near the ventrocaudal area of the fish through the anus, or empty into a cloaca that serves as a small vestibule for excretion of the digestive waste, urinary waste, and reproductive products through the vent.

Histology

The intestine consists of a mucosa, submucosa, muscularis, and serosa layers, although in many teleosts the muscularis is not present. The teleost intestine has many longitudinal folds to increase the absorptive surface area. The pyloric cecae and intestinal mucosa are composed of mucoid columnar epithelial cells that may have a brush border of microvilli, but few fish possess villae. The pyloric ceca do not typically contain cells that secrete digestive enzymes. There are numerous secreting rodlet and mucous cells. Many fish also have patches of lymphoid tissue. Submucosa of these organs contains smooth muscle, eosinophilic granular cells, and a fibroelastic area. When the muscularis is present it consists of circular and longitudinal smooth muscle. In cyprinids, striped or striated muscle can also be found in

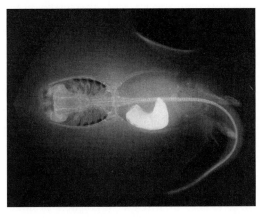

Fig. 1. A dorso-ventral (DV) radiograph of a clinically normal yellow stingray (*Urolophus jamaicensis*) given barium to visualize the spiral colon.

the intestinal mucosa. The rectum is highly distensible, muscular, and mucinogenic. Microvilli may be present on the rectoepithelial cells. Elasmobranchs also contain rectal glands that are believed to help in osmoregulation with sodium and chloride.

Physiologic considerations

The intestines are the site for continued chemical or enzymatic digestion and nutrient absorption. The pancreas produces many of the digestive enzymes, and the liver contributes bile for absorption in the small intestine. Nutrient absorption through the enterocytes can be active or passive with or without the use of carrier molecules. Some species of fish use microbial fermentation for digestion in their intestines. The intestines rely on smooth muscle contraction to keep the flow of digesta, and transit times vary greatly for fish species according to multiple dietary (herbivores verses carnivores) and environmental factors (water temperature).

Pancreas and liver

Anatomic considerations

The pancreas in fish may be a discrete organ, diffuse, or be part of the liver and referred to as a hepatopancreas. In certain species, discrete pancreatic material is often found in fat that surrounds the pyloric cecae. The main pancreatic duct usually empties into the common bile duct. The pancreas contains cells that produce both exocrine and endocrine products used for digestion.

The liver in most fish is found in the anterior abdomen, and is generally extremely large. Blood is provided via the hepatic artery and drains via one or multiple portal veins. In elasmobranchs, the liver can be as much as 25% of the body weight of certain species. Fish also have gall bladders, and gall can vary in color, having various shades of green, yellow, or brown. The liver itself can also vary in color, from deep reddish brown to pale yellow. The gall bladder empties via a bile duct into the pyloric region of the stomach and small intestine.

Histology

The pancreas contains both exocrine and endocrine components. Typical teleosts exocrine cells have zymogen granules, causing them to appear basophilic with staining. Ascini are formed by the pancreatic secretory cells with ducts that open into the intestine or intestinal ceca. Endocrine cells of the pancreas are large and granulated. Numerous endocrine islet cells have been described in a variety of species. Aggregates of endocrine cells have been referred to as Brockmann bodies. In fish, endocrine and exocrine cells are located in separate aggregates.

Histologically, the liver of fish differs from other vertebrates because chords and lobes are not as distinct, and the sinusoids have blood on one side and a bile channel on the opposite side. Hepatocytes of fish often contain substantial amounts of lipid and small amounts of ceroid [11]. Bile ducts originate intracellularly. The liver may also contain pancreatic tissue, melanomacrophage centers, and hematopoietic tissue. Hematopoietic tissue can sometimes be found in cuffs surrounding hepatic blood vessels. Depending on the fish species, either lipid-rich or glycogen-rich hepatocytes may predominate. This storage of lipid or glycogen can also be a function of diet, particularly in commercially raised or captive individuals. Functional Kupffer cells are found to line the sinusoids of many species. Fish also have fat storage cells called cells of Ito that are located in the space of Disse between the hepatocytes and sinusoidal cells. In elasmobranchs, fat vacuoles appear larger than in teleosts. Hepatocytes of fish can be swollen with glycogen even at times of marginal nutrition [13]. The gallbladder is cuboidal or columnar epithelium.

Physiologic considerations

Although the liver and pancreas function similar to other vertebrates, special considerations must be made when reviewing fish energy metabolism. Most species of fish have slow glucose metabolism and do not require rapid glucose homeostasis. Many fish can readily employ gluconeogenesis when carbohydrates are low. The pancreas uses both exocrine and endocrine peptides to facilitate digestion and energy metabolism similar to other vertebrates. Pancreatic islet cells have been identified as insulin, glucagons, or somatosin-secreting cells [14].

The primary function of the liver in teleosts is to conjugate bile. Unconjugated bilirubin that has been converted from hemoglobin from dying red cells in the reticuloendothelial system circulates in the blood and attaches to albumin. When unconjugated bilirubin enters the liver, glucuronic acid attaches to the bilirubin to form bilirubin diglucuronide in the hepatocytes. This conjugated product is excreted via the bile ducts to the gall bladder. The gall bladder secretes this bile into the intestines, where bile helps with fat breakdown for nutrient absorption in the intestines. In elasmobranchs, the liver produces squalene, which helps these animals maintain their buoyancy. Pancreatic products and bile produced by the liver are responsible for the final digestion and absorption of nutrients in the gastrointestinal system.

Swimbladder

Anatomic considerations

The swimbladder, although not a functional part of the alimentary tract, is derived from the digestive tract [15]. There is tremendous variability with swimbladders in fish, and many different strategies for maintaining buoyancy. Some species of fish, especially deep benthos animals, do not have any swimbladders or have lost their swimbladders. This organ resembles a balloon that lies along the dorsal peritoneal cavity just below the kidneys. This organ may run the entire length of the peritoneal cavity. As noted earlier, in some species of fish this organ is filled with air via a duct that opens into the esophagus. It may consist of one or two chambers (Fig. 2). Swimbladders with an esophageal opening are referred to as a physostomous swimbladder. In many species of fish this duct may not be present. Swimbladders without esophageal opening are physoclistic. These fish rely on anastomoses of blood vessels called the *rete mirabila* and gas gland to exchange gas across the swimbladder. Certain species of fish have developmental changes that employ strategies in which fry are physiosto-mous and must fill their swimbladders shortly after hatching, but as maturing to adults these fry lose this esophageal connection or even the entire swimbladder at latter developmental stages.

Histology

The swimbladder forms from the foregut in fish. Most fish swimbladders consist of a tunica externa and tunica interna. The serosal tunica externa consists of fibrous connective tissue, muscle, and elastic tissue. The mucosa of the tunica interna, which lines the gas space, has a submucosal area of loose vascular connective tissue, a muscularis mucosa, and transitional epithelium [10].

Physiologic considerations

The swimbladder has several functions. The primary function is for buoyancy, which is controlled by swallowing or belching air for physostomus species, and gas exchange via arterial plexus and gas gland for emptying and

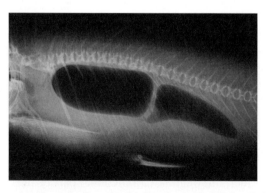

Fig. 2. A lateral radiograph of a normal inflated swimbladder in a koi (*C carpio*).

filling this organ in physoclistic species. The swimbladder is used for sound and pressure detection in some species. Sea ravens (*Hemitripterus americanus*) use their swimbladder to produce sounds, possibly for courtship.

The piscine diagnostic workup

When aquarists at the NEAq suspect a health problem with an individual or group of animals, they contact the Animal Health Department. If the animal is large enough, and capture can be readily facilitated, a full clinical workup is performed. The procedures for a typical veterinary examination are outlined below, with reference to specific presentations that may be encountered with animals that have gastrointestinal problems.

Water chemistry and history

Before beginning any clinical workup, water chemistry is performed on the tank environment to check for a variety of physical and chemical factors. These tests are performed to make sure that adequate oxygen is available, there is not a significant waste accumulation in the tank, and also to ensure that optimum requirements are being maintained for this particular species. On occasion, special testing may be requested for either microbiologic testing or heavy metal testing.

The veterinary staff also obtains a history from aquarist staff most familiar with this animal. Often times in public aquaria several types of histories are gathered. The natural history of the specific species is readily obtained from knowledgeable aquarists and also researched via present literature. Natural history can offer significant insight regarding behavior, habitat, diet, reproduction, and water-quality parameters. This knowledge is extremely vital for rare or exotic species that may not afford substantial clinical baseline data following the physical examination.

Exhibit history is also obtained, which entails understanding any changes to the exhibit or changes in water-quality parameters. Many physical and chemical changes can be garnered from an exhibit history such as lighting changes; temperature changes; life-support failures, adjustments or alterations; stocking densities; new introductions; intra- or interspecific aggression; and feeding schedules.

A behavioral/husbandry history for the individual animal includes information about how this animal has typically behaved and thrived. These questions for the individual history will lead to the animal's present health. Some questions include: How is the animal behaving? What does the animal eat? What is the feeding frequency? How are other tank mates? Are any other animals exhibiting abnormal behavior? When were the problems first noted? How long has the animal been in captivity?

The medical history is obtained when gathering information for the individual animal. Often, there may be significant deviations from natural history verses captivity; but if an animal has thrived for several years in the exhibit, some natural history concerns may become less relevant.

Physical examination

After taking a good history and checking water-quality parameters, the patient is then ready for a physical examination. First the animal is observed in the exhibit, and behavior, body condition, color, and respirations are noted. Often, if the animal is not eating, the animal is observed during a scheduled feeding time. This can help to distinguish animals that are not interested in food or acclimating to captivity verses animals that are trying to eat but may be unable because of several factors such as intra- or interspecies aggression, traumatic injury to the mouth or jaw, wrong food type, and/or many other reasons. Body condition can be determined quite readily, although in some of the laterally compressed species this may be difficult to fully assess. When assessing body condition, one should look at both the abdominal area and also along the spine [16]. If the animal has been anorexic for a short time, the dorsal musculature may not be affected even though the animal may have a thin abdomen. Wasting along the spine indicates more of a chronic condition that may focus on other questions. Is the animal eating but not able to gain weight or is the animal anorectic?

If the animals are over 50 g, anesthesia is performed using a water-soluble anesthetic agent in tank water for this species. The animals then undergo a physical examination, weight, caudal vein phlebotomy for a complete blood cell count and blood chemistry, a fecal swab and fecal examination, a cloacal lavage, skin and gill biopsy for microscopy, and radiography as standard procedures at NEAq.

The gastrointestinal patient

During the physical examination briefly highlighted above, information is often gathered that may suggest gastrointestinal problems. This information may lead to further diagnostics or be sufficient to begin a treatment.

History, physical examination, and weight

From the history and physical exam, information may lead to a differential diagnosis list that suggests gastrointestinal disease. Some important information includes animal nutrition, feeding behavior, and overall appearance/body condition. Nutrition has been studied in depth for many of the commercially valuable species, with several textbooks available on this topic alone. Some pathologic conditions caused by nutritional problems are found in Halver's fish nutrition [17]. Body condition and abdominal appearance can discern an animal that is chronically wasting away verses an animal that may be acutely anorexic, as previously noted [16]. An animal with abdominal distension needs to be further evaluated to distinguish fat, gonads, foreign body, neoplasia, or ascites. Extreme ascites in many species may cause the scales to rise, giving the animal a pinecone appearance. A proper weight on a fish is necessary to provide proper doses for certain treatments, and monitor mass and fluid loss or gain.

Complete blood cell count and blood chemistry screen

For most species of fish in the public aquarium setting, baseline normal values for blood do not exist, except for the most commercially important species. For some of the more commonly seen teleost species and for several elasmobranchs, Stoskopf has published some baseline data in the text *Fish Medicine* [16]. Unfortunately, most baseline data remain inaccessible for veterinarians because it exists as unpublished research, medical notes, and medical records in many public aquaria. The complete blood cell count is extremely valuable for identifying infections, erythrocyte perturbations, and protein loss [2]. Identifying different leukocytes in teleosts and elasmobranchs can be quite challenging, and often requires regular practice of laboratory technicians or hematologists trained specifically for aquatic animals. Blood chemistry screens in fish have some value as well. To evaluate hepatic disease, alanine aminotransferase, aspartate aminotransferase, and bile acids can be taken. At NEAq, sudden increases in these enzymes have been associated with acute septicemia and hepatitis in several teleost species. As with higher vertebrates, the values for these enzymes must be placed in context of the animal's history and clinical condition. High or low values for any serum chemistry parameters must be carefully evaluated and acted upon cautiously, because high or low values are often not specific for individual disease problems. Animals with significant liver or gastrointestinal disease may have "normal" serum chemistry values, when evaluated.

Fecal analysis/cloacal lavage

Fecal analysis in fish is similar to other animals using standard fecal flotation techniques. Many of the common parasites can often be identified to genus and species and treatments initiated. Cestodes, trematodes, and nematodes are all common findings in fish, with cestodes and nematodes commonly found in the feces. Often slides are made from fecal swabs using a diff quick and acid-fast staining technique to evaluate bacterial flora, and to determine if animals are shedding acid-fast bacteria. In addition to metazoan pathogens and mycobacteria detection, cloacal lavage with sterile saline and a sterile French catheter are a means to better identify some of the protozoan pathogens in the gastrointestinal tract of fish. Different coccidial species have been identified in clinically ill and healthy animals using this technique in teleost and elasmobranchs. This may also prove beneficial to identify flagellate protozoans that are hexamita-like.

Peritoneal washes or lavages are used regularly in rays to check for coccidian infection. These washes are generally done using a sterile needle, syringe, and saline. Samples can be examined under light microscopy and cultured. These washes are ultrasound guided to avoid accidentally perforating any organs of the alimentary tract.

Diagnostic imaging

Radiography, ultrasonography, and CT scans can be easily done in fish. Radiography has limitations in viewing soft tissue, but with barium contrast either orally or per vent or rectum, the gastrointestinal tract can be readily viewed (Fig. 3A and B). This technique is particularly helpful to distinguish abdominal masses from either gastrointestinal or reproductive tissue origin. At the NEAq, fish are frequently ultrasounded for abdominal distention to distinguish ascites from gonads or other masses. Ultrasonagraphy can be done on an unanesthetized animal. The probe is protected from water using a plastic rectal sleeve. The water helps eliminate air that may be trapped in and around the various scale patterns of individual species. Biopsies or peritoneal fluid can be readily obtained using ultrasound in piscine patients. CT scans offer the greatest prospects for soft tissue evaluation, and can specifically delineate masses in the abdomen.

Endoscopy and surgery

Endoscopy and exploratory surgery are also used in aquatic animal medicine for fish. Laparoscopy is used for abdominal exploration and organ biopsies. Exploratory or general surgery may be required for mass removal or, as a final option, for diagnosis and/or treatment. For more information on fish surgery, one can read Harms and Lewbart [5]. As endoscopy/

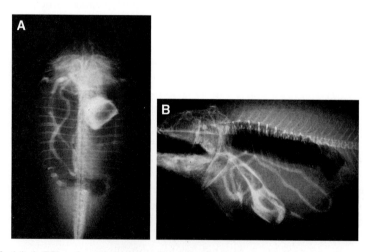

Fig. 3. (*A*) A DV and a (*B*) lateral radiograph of a barium contrast study shows a mass (lipoma) intertwined in the gastrointestinal tract of a large-mouth bass (*Micropterus salmonides*).

laparoscopy becomes a more readily available option for aquatic animal veterinarians, this equipment will be extremely helpful for diagnosing several common disease problems and performing treatments or surgery in the piscine abdomen.

Gastrointestinal diseases in fish

Mycobacteriosis

Aquatic species of mycobacteria have been investigated for years, but since 1999, this pathogen has become a more significant factor in emerging diseases for aquatic animal professionals [18]. Several species of mycobacteria can infect fish and cause granulomatous disease in these animals [19]. Mycobacteriosis in fish is of particular concern because it is a zoonotic pathogen, and because recent outbreaks have been found in commercially important wild populations and aquaculture-reared animals [20–22]. Mycobacteriosis can clinically manifest itself in a variety of ways. Cases can range from vague to classic presentations of the disease. Some clinical cases are described below.

A blue tang (*Acanthurus coeruleus*) presented with difficulty maintaining posture. The animal was unable to lift its caudal fin. Diagnostic testing showed the animal had a slightly elevated white blood cell count. Radiographs showed severe spinal damage with bony remodeling along the caudal third of the spine and a mass in the caudal portion of the peritoneal cavity (Fig. 4). The animal was euthanized due to a poor prognosis, and mycobacterial granulomas were through the gastrointestinal tract and along the spinal column. The mass was a 5 cm-diameter mycobacterial granuloma.

Twenty scad (*Selar crumenophthalmus*) presented with thin body condition, and a few individuals had some skin lesions. Acid-fast slides were positive from skin lesion biopsies. Because these animals were in quarantine, euthanasia was elected. Ten of 20 animals cultured positive for *Mycobacterium fortuitum* from cultures obtained from the alimentary tract.

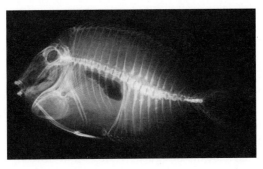

Fig. 4. A lateral radiograph of a blue tang (*A coeruleus*) showing severe bony changes of the spine caused by mycobacteriosis.

A pet Siamese fighting fish (*Beta splendis*) presented with poor coloration, thin body condition, and missing scales in the pectoral region. The animal was eating well. The animal died after initial presentation, and mycobacteria was confirmed on necropsy, cultured from several gastrointestinal granulomas.

Other signs attributed to mycobacteriosis in fish include reproductive problems, oral masses [23], head swelling, exophthalmia, coelomic distention, opercular masses skin lesions, poor growth, emaciation with or without anorexia, nonhealing skin ulcers, exophthalmia, and swimming or postural deficits often associated with skeletal abnormalities [24]. Many times clinical signs are not present, and mycobacteriosis is found on postmortem examination.

Diagnosis

Mycobacteriosis can be caused by several species of mycobacteria that are prevalent in aquatic environments. These bacteria are acid-fast staining, using Ziehl-Nielson stains [25]. In the public aquaria setting, diagnosis of mycobacteriosis may be made on clinical presentation with confirmation of acid-fast organisms from lesions or granulomas. Mycobacteriosis can then be definitively confirmed using microbiologic testing, but culture and isolation can require several weeks for this organism to grow. Several researchers are trying to develop polymerase chain reaction and enzyme-linked immunosorbent assays tests for fish for faster diagnosis (personal communication with Dr. Salvatore Frasca, University of Connecticut, Department of Pathobiology) [26,27].

Treatment

Clinical treatment for fish has not been greatly successful, although some combination of antibacterial therapies have been tried in several species [28]. Conroy and Conroy [29] reported successful treatment using the amino-glycoside, Kanamycin, regimen in fancy veiled tail guppies, but this treatment has not provided the same results in other species at NEAq. The unreliability of antemortem diagnostic testing for mycobacteria prevents thorough evaluation of treatment efficacy. Because this disease can cause a zoonotic infection, commonly referred to as fish handler's disease, treatment options should be carefully planned and executed if attempted to prevent spreading the infection to other tanks and to ensure staff safety. The tenacity of aquatic species of mycobacteria to survive also suggests that with multiple treatment regimes antibiotic resistance can develop similar to the resistance already prevalent with mammalian and avian strains of tuberculosis. Recombinant DNA vaccines are being designed, tested, and investigated to prevent infection of fish from mycobacteriosis, yet these vaccines have not provided a protective response against challenge infection [30,31].

Studies in zebra fish models for mycobacteriosis may offer hope for a broader understanding of fish immune response and protection to this disease [32]. Mycobacterial infections and outbreaks are being investigated in clinically ill striped bass (*Morone saxatilis*) from wild populations in the Chesapeake Bay, which, as a wild infection, may pose quarantine, human safety, and collection management dilemmas for public aquaria that collect native species on a regular basis. Research is progressing toward the development of nonlethal and inexpensive testing methods for *Mycobacteria* sp. that would strengthen quarantine antemortem screening for potentially infected animals. Based on all these factors, mycobacteriosis is a disease that is best managed by prevention through the development of proper quarantine, sanitation, habitat optimization, and nutrition and disinfection programs.

Infectious pancreatic necrosis

Infectious pancreatic necrosis (IPN) is caused by a birnavirus, and is one of the most widely distributed aquatic animal viruses in the world. It primarily has affected salmonid commercial aquaculture, but it can infect several other fish species. Clinical signs noted below can be pathognomonic for disease in salmonids, and mortality and infection can be influenced by temperature. At high temperatures (10–14°C) mortality can be rapid and quite high, while at temperatures lower than 10°C overall mortalities can be low, but occur over a longer time period [33]. This disease causes catarrhal enteritis in salmonids, causing high mortalities in young fish. Animals often darken, and may have unilateral or bilateral exophthalmia, abdominal distension, and are trailing pale fecal casts. Necropsy commonly reveals pale organs, ascites, and gastrointestinal petechiae. On histology, infected individuals exhibit focal necrosis of acinar pancreatic tissue. Lidipose cells surrounding pancreatic tissue may also be necrotic. Animals may be asymptomatic carriers of the disease.

Diagnosis

Diagnosis can be based on clinical signs for most commercially raised salmonids with laboratory confirmation. Because this is a significant concern for commercial aquaculture, postmortem testing is readily available and rapid. IPN virus can be identified in tissues using indirect fluorescent antibody testing. Enzyme-linked immunosorbent assays detect virus in the serum. Virus isolation followed with cytopathic effect and serum neutralization testing is available for IPN. A caveat for interpreting any positive test results for IPN is that animals can be subclinical carriers.

Treatment

There is no treatment for fish infected with IPN. In many states and countries, IPN is considered a reportable disease that may lead to stringent depopulation and disinfection protocols for infected farms. Proper management that includes disinfection, quarantine, and broodstock testing on a regular basis is the best method to avoid having fish infected with IPN. Many producers require that stocking fry come from IPN free farms and broodstock. Many producers may even require fry be tested before shipment for stocking. Although vaccine protection has been promising for IPN, crossprotection has not been found with the numerous serotypes of virus infecting commercial populations.

Coccidiosis

Coccidia are intracellular protozoans. The identification of coccidian species in pokilotherms has greatly expanded in recent years [34]. Steve Uptown, at Kansas State University, has identified several species of coccidia in teleost fish and elasmobranchs [35–38]. The importance of coccidia causing enteritis in wild and captive fish populations continues to be investigated. Previous health investigations in two wild dogfish species found coccidia as one of several potentially pathogenic organisms present in animals with multiple gastric lesions, although coccidia's pathologic significance in these animals could not be distinguished from other pathogens found [39]. In public aquaria, coccidian infections have been associated with enteritis and peritonitis in elasmobranchs [40] and sygnathids [38].

In one of the first reported outbreaks in cownose rays (*Rhinoptera bonasus*), animals became emaciated and developed coelomic ascites. In these animals oocysts were not found in the feces [41]. Clinical infection may be asymptomatic. In clinically affected sharks and rays at NEAq, the animals often abruptly stop feeding. Some animals may have blackened feces from digested blood or sloughed intestinal epithelium. Sometimes animals may appear thin, and sudden death in rays has occurred. Rays and sharks that develop clinical signs have also been exposed to other stressors. Some examples including transport, aggression resulting in bites (even superficial rakes), poor water quality, low dissolved oxygen, or medical bath treatments with chemicals such as copper sulfate. Copper sulfate is not widely used or recommended with elasmobranchs, but in public aquaria with dynamic exhibitry, copper treatment may be warranted to preserve valuable collections that contain both teleosts and elasmobranchs during specific disease outbreaks.

Diagnosis

Oocystes can be identified using coelomic cavity aspirate sampling [42]. Oocyts have also been identified from a cloacal wash or fecal analysis, but oocyst presence alone does not signify an infection, and these findings should be correlated with clinical presentation.

Treatment

Several coccidiostats are available and have been used in fish at varying dosages. Diclazuril, totrazuril, and sulfadimidine have been used as oral and bath treatments in elamobranchs [41]. Stamper reported a dosage of 10 mg toltrazuril/kg orally once a day for 5 days reduced clinical signs in cownose rays [42]. With elasmobranchs, stress should be minimized and water quality parameters optimized.

Enteric septicemia of catfish

Enteric septicemia of catfish (ESC) is common in commercially raised channel catfish (*Ictalarus punctatus*), caused by a Gram-negative bacterium called *Edwardsiella ictaluri*. ESC in channel catfish may present with clinical signs or manifest as acute mortality. There are acute and chronic forms of the disease that are related to route of exposure via the gastrointestinal tract or olfactory organ, respectively [43]. Fish sometimes will abruptly go off feed. Fish may be seen swimming at the surface listlessly, appearing to drag their caudal fin, or swim in a corkscrew pattern. When fish are examined, they may have small circular skin ulcerations over the body, ulcerations over the skull, abdominal extension, or exophthalmia. The hole in the head lesion in channel catfish is considered pathognomonic for ESC. ESC infection and mortality is temperature dependent, occurring in late spring and fall in the southeastern United States.

Diagnosis

Diagnosis for ESC is commonly made with microbiology, and the organism can grow within 24 hours using tryptic soy or brain–heart infusion agars. Often, based on clinical signs and positive culture results, treatment is initiated. Enzyme-linked immunosorbent assay is also available for more rapid diagnosis.

Treatment

Vaccines are currently being tested and developed for this pathogen. Treatments include medicated feeds that contain either oxytetracycline or ormetoprim–sulfadimethoxine. Typical treatment for disease outbreaks requires quick diagnosis because the catfish will typically go off feed shortly after infection. As with all agricultural disease outbreaks, husbandry and environmental conditions should also be investigated to decrease stress for commercial ponds.

Cestodes (tapeworms) and nematodes (roundworms)

There are numerous cestodes and nematodes that can infect fish. Often fish do not show clinical signs. The most common clinical signs are weight loss despite good appetite. Sometimes worms can be seen passing through the anus or vent. One cestode of particular importance is the Asian tapeworm (*Bothriocephalus acheilognathi*). This worm was introduced from China in imported grass carp (*Ctenopharyngodon idellus*). It poses particular risk because it can infect a wide range of hosts, including koi, carp species, baitfish, and freshwater aquarium species. In several states and countries infection with this parasite is reportable.

Nematodes are commonly found in fish. In some species of aquarium fish, nematodes may cause reproductive problems, slow growth, or a failure to thrive. In public aquarium, species with the highest infection of nematodes include species that are typically benthic like the walking batfish (*Ogcocephalus vespertilio*). In this species, heavy infections can cause significant mortalities in captivity.

Diagnosis

Both groups of parasites can be identified via fecal examination and float, with either worms, proglottids, or eggs being identified for cestodes and nematodes. When performing health examinations, gastrointestinal wet mounts can be used for Asian tapeworm infection.

Treatment

For both cestodes and nematodes, basic husbandry practices that use prepared rather than live food sources can greatly decrease parasite load for many species. Antihelmenthics can be used orally for treatment. For cestodes, praziquantel is commonly used. Nematodes can be treated with a variety of drugs. Fenbendazole and levamasole are commonly used. Ivermectin has a low therapeutic index in some species of fish and should be used with caution [6]. Because Asian tapeworm infection is reportable in some states and countries, infection with this parasite may have greater implications for depopulation and disinfection on fish farms.

Nutrition problems—fatty liver syndrome

Hepatic lipidosis or fatty liver syndrome can occur in fish. This often is an incidental finding for collection fish or may present as acute mortality in commercial fish. It is often diagnosed on necropsy, but could be found with liver biopsy or other diagnostic imaging tools. Often animals diagnosed in the collection at postmortem are geriatric animals that are overweight and have been feed heavily to avoid predation. These animals are usually target fed specific diets on exhibit, but also have some access to indiscriminate broadcast feeding for other species. In commercial aquaculture, large-mouth bass from some farms were found to have hepatic lipidosis after experiencing some acute mortalities. The etiology of this syndrome in young large-mouth bass (*Micropterus salmonides*), was hypothesized as too high carbohydrate levels in commercial feed for this species [44]. Optimizing nutrition for these animals can prevent associated nutritional problems [45].

Dysphagia

Fish in public aquaria have been known to ingest various foreign bodies accidentally or on purpose. These objects have included items dropped in exhibits by the public, normal habitat items, and items used by aquarists. Some items have included rubber balls, plastic animals, stones, food sticks, lead weights, air stones, and tank mates. If these incidents are discovered early, often items or other fish can be removed nonsurgically, and both prey and predator saved (Fig. 5A and 5B).

Spironucleus, cryptobia, and hexamita species

Small flagellated protozoa [46] have been identified as causing enteritis and gastroenteritis in a variety of commercial and aquarium trade fish. In

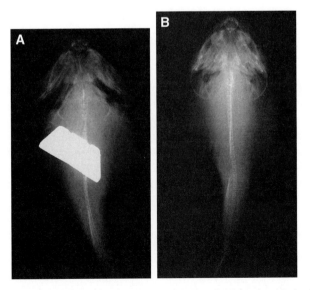

Fig. 5. (*A*) A DV radiograph of a sea raven (*H americanus*) after ingestion of a lead weight and air tubing. (*B*) A DV radiograph of a sea raven (*H americanus*) after manual removal of ingested lead weight and air tubing.

1974, the National Veterinary Institute in Norway identified hexamitid flagellates using light microscopy as the etiology for catarrhal enteritis in brown trout (*Salmo trutta*). Spironucleaus outbreaks have been implicated for significant economic losses in commercial aquaculture for several species, causing systemic infections in sea-caged salmon (*Salmo salar*) [47,48]. Another species of flagellated protozoa, *Cryptobia iublans*, caused an outbreak of systemic disease in African cichlids at the Shedd Aquarium in Chicago causing 50% mortality [49].

Fish develop signs associated with enteric disease, often resulting in loss of appetite. Because catarrhal enteritis may develop, anemia may occur. Ascites, which may or may not be accompanied with abdominal distension, is common in infected animals. Fish may then waste away, or, with chronic infections, animals may fail to thrive.

Diagnosis

Motile trophozoites can be identified using light microscopy and dark field on intestinal contents, fecal analysis, or cloacal lavage. On postmortem, organisms can be generally identified through wet mounts of the gastrointestinal tract, especially of stomach or intestinal granulomas. These granulomas most be differentiated from other etiologies that include fungi, mycobacteria, streptococci, and metazoan parasites. Many species of hexamita-like flagellated protozoans may be difficult to see using light microscopy. Definitive species identification must be completed using electron microscopy. Electron microscopy has been used to help ultrastructurally identify spironucleus infections in burbot (*Lota lota*) [50], salmonids, and grayling [51].

Treatment/control

Because these outbreaks infect both commercial food and aquarium fish, treatment is riddled with several problems that include application, efficacy, and drug withdrawal times in certain captive situations. Antiflagellate medications, like metronidazole, have been reported efficacious, although healthy fish are known to carry hexamita species [52]. As with any disease outbreak in fish systems, the best method of treatment is prevention. If an outbreak occurs, review of water quality, husbandry, quarantine, nutrition, and sanitation is warranted to optimize environmental conditions.

Piscine gastrointestinal differential diagnosis

Gastroenterology in teleost fish [53–60] and elasmobranchs poses many challenges. The diversity of fish species provides different anatomic, histologic, and physiologic variations and adaptations, which have evolved to accommodate for diverse and harsh aquatic environments from the artic depths to desert puddles. As in higher vertebrates, veterinary diagnostic and

Table 1
Piscine gastrointestinal differential diagnosis

Gastrointestinal tract	Etiology	Diseases/problems	Common name/misc
Mouth/oral cavity	*Infectious*		
	Viral	Lymphocystis (iridoviris)	Can infect dermal fibroblast cells of lips
		Angel cichlid fibroma	
		Oncorhynchus masu virus (OMV)	May be of retroviral origin Survivors can develop epithelial tumors of mouth.
	Bacterial	*Yersinia ruckeri*	Enteric red mouth
		Cytophaga Columnaris	columnaris
		Cytophaga-like	Cotton mouth
		Pseudomonas anguilliseptical	Sekiten-byo; petechia around mouth, operculum and ventrum
	Fungal	Several species	Ulcers, dermal masses, fluffy tufts on the lips and mouth
	Metazoan	*Bucephalus polymorphus*	
	Noninfectious		
	Neoplasia	Squamous cell carcinoma	Can affect oral cavity
		Stomatopapilloma	Mouth growths
		Gilthead sea bream papilloma	Maxillary tumors
	Traumatic	Broken jaw, loose or missing teeth, unable to close lips or mouth	Handling, aggression, habitat problems, dysphagia (ie pebbles) Jaw fractures can heal.
Esophagus	*Infectious*		
	Protozoan	*Heterosporis finki*	Infects esophagus muscle of freshwater angelfish
	Metazoan	Encysted or migrating nematodes	Clinically important in large numbers
		Encysted digenian metacercariae	Often secondary finding on pathology
	Noninfectious		
	Foreign bodies	Fin spines, artificial habitat, fish hooks	Can be surgically or manually removed
	Neoplasia	Striated muscle	
	Myopathies	Striated muscle or circular muscle problems	
Stomach	*Infectious*		
	Bacterial	*Mycobacteria* spp (multiple)	Very common, no treatment, and zoonotic
		Nocardia asteroids	Clinically similar to mycobacteriosis

(*continued on next page*)

Table 1 (*continued*)

Gastrointestinal tract	Etiology	Diseases/problems	Common name/misc
	Fungal	*Saprolegnia* spp	
	Protozoans	Myxozoans—*Myxobolus dermatobia; M exiguus*	Associated with mass mortalities
		Microsporidians—*glugea* spp	
		Haemagregarine sachai	
		Flagellates—*Cryptobia* spp; *Hexamita-like* spp; *Spironucleus*	Causes gastric granulomas
	Metazoans	*Anasakis* spp	Gadoid fishes and zoonotic
		Cestode spp	Most often metazoans are
		Nematode spp	an incidental finding in
		Acanthocephalan spp	most fishes and clinically
		Digenean trematode spp	relevant in large numbers.
	Noninfectious		
	Toxins	Noxious algae	
		Bufo marinus—marine toad	Reported to cause hemorrhagic gastritis in sharks after ingestion
	Water Quality	Nephrocalcinosis	Calcified granulomas in stomach mucosa
	Misc.	Atrophy associated with sexual maturity	
		Ingestion of foreign objects and fish hooks	Can be removed manually, with endoscopy, and/or gastrotomy
Intestinal	*Infectious*		
	Viral	Infectious pancreatic necrosis (IPN)	Pyloric cecae McKnight cells swell and fragment nucleus.
		Infectious hematopoietic necrosis (IHN)	Eosinophilic granular cell necrosis of intestine
		Viral hemorrhagic septicemia (VHS)	Primary kidney pathogen with secondary intestinal hemorrhage and necrosis
		Channel catfish viral disease adenovirus (CCVD)	Intestinal necrosis Intestinal and spiral valve epithelial cells swell.
		Retrovirus	
		Spring viremia of carp (SVC)	Enteritis

Table 1 (*continued*)

Gastrointestinal tract	Etiology	Diseases/problems	Common name/misc
	Bacterial	*Mycobacteria* spp	Granulomatous disease
		Vibrio spp	
		Aeromonas salmonicida	
		Edwardsiella ictaluri	
		Yersinia ruckeri	
		Streptococcus spp	*Streptococcus* spp can cause granulomas; serosanguinous fluid in intestines and peritoneal cavity
	Fungal	*Icthyophonus hoferi*	
		Phoma herbarum	
	Protozoan	Microsporidians—*Glugea stephani; Glugea* spp;	*G Stephani* can cause xenomas in intestinal connective tissue of flatfishes.
		Entrocytozoan salmonis	
		Myxozoans—*Thelhanellus kitauei; Myxidium giardi*	
		Coccidia—*Eimeria* spp;	
		Epieimeria spp; *Goussia* spp; *Calptospora* spp	
		Crytosporidia spp	
		Flagellates—*Hexamita* spp;	
		Cryptobia iubilans;	Hexamita-like organisms
		Spironucleus spp	can cause intestinal necrosis and granulomas.
	Metazoan	*Acanthocephalus* spp	Some species are zoonotic.
		Bothriocephalus spp	Mainly incidental
		Eubothrim spp	findings on necropsy
		Diphyllobothrim spp	
	Noninfectious		
	Heavy metals	Pb, Cd	
	Toxins	Blue Green algae	Can cause intussusception
Pancreas	*Infectious*		
	Viral	IPN	Necrosis of pancreatic
		PD	acinar cells
		IHN	Pancreatic necrosis
		Eel Birnaviruses	IPN-like
		Herpesvirus salmonis	Symptoms similar to IPN Pathognomonic: pancreatic syncytia
	Bacterial	Multiple	
	Noninfectious		
	Idiopathic	Pancreas disease	Affects sea-cultured salmonids and is marked by pancreatic necrosis
	Nutritional	Pansteatitis	

(*continued on next page*)

Table 1 (*continued*)

Gastrointestinal tract	Etiology	Diseases/problems	Common name/misc
Liver	*Infectious*		
	Viral	IHN	Hepatic necrosis
		CCVD	Necrosis
		Focal necrotizing hepatitis	Some focal hepatic necrosis
		Reovirus	
		Rhabdoviral salmonid hepatitis	Hepatitis
	Bacterial	*Aeromonas salmonicida*	Necrosis and hemorrhage
		Renibacterium salmonarum	Hepatic granulomas
		Staphyloccus aureus	*S aureus* was identified as a cause of liver granulomas in two smooth dogfish (*Mustelus canis*) in a touch tank exhibit.
	Fungal	*Ichthyophonus* spp	
		Exophilia spp	
	Protozoal	*Myxidium* spp—*Chloromyxum truttae;*	*Can cause pseudocysts* *C truttae infects gallbladder and bile ducts*
		Ceratomyxa Shasta	
		Hexamita spp	
		Coccidia—Goussia clupearum; Goussia metchnikovi	Necrosis, hepatitis, fibrosis and white or black foci on liver
	Metazoal	*Trianophorus* spp	
	Noninfectious		
	Nutritional	Rancid fat—fatty liver ceroidosis	
		Gallstones	
	Toxins	Aflatoxins—*Aspergillus flavus*	Many heavy toxins can cause focal hepatic necrosis, while herbicides and pesticides may induce hepatic neoplasia.
		Anoxia	
		Cd, Hg, PCBs	
		Pb, Cu, Al, Zn	
		Algal toxins	Hepatorenal syndrome in turbot with Pb in diet
	Neoplasia	Toxin induced	
Swimbladder	*Infectious*		
	Viral	*Rhabdovirus carpio*	Inflammation and hemorrhage
	Bacterial	*Actinobacter-like*	Swimbladder hemorrhage
	Fungal	*Phoma herbarum*	Can implicate poorly sanitized hatcheries
	Protozoal	Myxozoans—*Sphaerospora renicola*	Inflammation
		Coccidia—Goussia gadi; Goussia cichlidarum	

Table 1 (*continued*)

Gastrointestinal tract	Etiology	Diseases/problems	Common name/misc
	Noninfectious		
	Trauma	Sudden pressure changes overfill swimbladder	Many spp of fish by catch brought up to water surface too quickly
	Idiopathethic	Swimbladder stress syndrome	Artic char
		Swimbladder filling problems	Fancy goldfish
		Improperly inflated swimbladders	Certain fish fry must gulp air to inflate swimbladders, and deficiencies of inflation have lead to negative buoyancy when rearing sygnathids.
Peritoneum	*Infectious*		
	Viral	Spring viremia of carp (SVC)	Peritonitis
	Bacterial	*Actinobacter-like*	Peritoneal hemorrhage
		Edwardsiella tarda	Postspawning fish; large
		Renibacterium salmonarum	amount of abdominal
		Lactobacillus spp— (Pseudokidney disease)	ascites *Streptococcus* spp can cause granulomas;
		Streptococcus spp	serosanguinous fluid in
		Vibrio spp	intestines and peritoneal cavity
	Fungal	*Phoma herbarum*	
		Exophila spp	
	Protozoal	*Eimeria* spp	Cow nosed rays
	Metazoal	*Ligula* spp	
		Diphyllobothrium spp	
	Noninfectious		
	Iatrogenic	Stripping of eggs; IP injections	Commercial salmonids
	Idiopathic	Systemic granuloma/ visceral granuloma/ Malawi bloat	Multiple visceral granulomas sometimes associated with calcium deposits; salmonids, seabream, African rift lake cichlids
	Miscellaneous	Gastrointestinal neoplasia	Ameloblastoma

This table is modified from work originally produced by Dr. Jimmy Turnbull. Modifications are supported with information from several current, respected, and expansive fish disease references.

Data from Refs [53–60].

treatment principles can be readily used to diagnose problems or diseases of the gastrointestinal tract in fish (Table 1). With a systematic approach, many gastrointestinal diseases in fish can be diagnosed and treated effectively. The current challenges found in aquatic animal medicine offers a field that will provide exciting fabric for establishing fish medicine as a desirable and practical veterinary specialty.

Acknowledgments

This article is dedicated to the Animal Health Department staff at the New England Aquarium. Dr. Tobias Schwartz provided digital copies of all the radiographs taken, and assisted with radiology for the gastrointestinal lipoma case. Dr. Tobias Schwartz, Lecturer in Veterinary Radiology, Department of Clinical Studies, School of Veterinary Medicine, University of Pennsylvania, 3850 Spruce Street, Philadelphia, PA 19104-6010.

References

[1] Nelson JS. Fishes of the world. 3rd edition. New York: John Wiley and Sons; 1994.
[2] Groff J, Zinkl J. Hematology and clinical chemistry of cyprinid fish: common carp and goldfish. In: Reavil DR, editor. Vet Clin North Am Exot Anim Pract 1999;2(3):741–76.
[3] Yanong RPE. Nutrition of ornamental fish. In: Jenkins JR, editor. Vet Clin North Am Exot Anim Pract 1999;2(1):19–42.
[4] Groff JM. Neoplasia in fishes. In: Graham JE, editor. Vet Clin North Am Exotic Anim Pract 2004;7(3): 705–56.
[5] Harms C, Lewbart G. Surgery in fish. In: Bennett RA, editor. Vet Clin North Am Exot Anim Pract 2000;3(3):759–74.
[6] Mashima T, Lewbart G. Pet fish formulary. In: Fronefield SA, editor. Vet Clin North Am Exot Anim Pract 2000;3(1):117–30.
[7] Bond CE. General morphology. In: Biology of fishes. 2nd edition. Orlando (FL): Saunders College Publishing; 1996. p. 15–56.
[8] Hanken J, Hall B, editors. The skulls. Volumes 1–3. Chicago: University of Chicago Press; 1993.
[9] Evans HE. Anatomy of tropical fishes. In: Gratzek JB, Matthews JR, editors. Aquariology: the science of fish health management (master volume). Morris Plains (NJ): Tetra Press; 1992. p. 71–94.
[10] Roberts RJ. The anatomy and physiology of teleosts. In: Fish pathology. 3rd edition. London: WB Saunders; 2001. p. 13–52.
[11] Ferguson HW. Systemic pathology of fish. Ames (IA): Iowa State Press; 1989.
[12] Fange R, Grove D. Digestion. In: Hoar WS, Randall DJ, Brett JR, editors. Fish physiology. Volume VIII: bioenergetics and growth. New York: Academic Press; 1979. p. 162–260.
[13] Horn MH. Feeding and digestion. In: Evans DH, editor. The physiology of fishes. 2nd edition. Boca Raton (FL): CRC Press; 1998. p. 43–64.
[14] Epple A. The endocrine pancreas. In: Hoar WS, Randall DJ, Brett JR, editors. Fish physiology Volume VIII: bioenergetics and growth. New York: Academic Press; 1969. p. 275–321.
[15] Stoskopf MK. Fish medicine. Philadelphia: WB Saunders; 1993. p. 2–30.
[16] Stoskopf MK. Fish medicine. Philadelphia: WB Saunders; 1993. p. 626.

[17] Roberts RJ, Bullock AM. The nutritional pathology of fishes. In: Halver JE, editor. Fish nutrition. London: Academic Press; 1989. p. 423–73.

[18] Austin B. Emerging bacterial fish pathogens. Bull Eur Assoc Fish Pathol 1999;19:231–4.

[19] Falkinham III, Joseph O. Epidemiology of infection by nontuberculous mycobacteria. Clin Microbiol Rev 1996;9:177–215.

[20] Dos Santos NMS, doVale A, Sousa MJ, et al. Mycobacterial infection in farmed turbot *Scophthalmus maximus*. Dis Aquat Organ 2003;52(1):87–91.

[21] Rhodes MW, Kator H, Kotob S, et al. *Mycobacterium shottsii* sp. nov., a slowly growing species isolated from Chesapeake Bay striped bass (*Morone saxatilis*). Int J Syst Evolut Microbiol 2003;53(2):421–4.

[22] Heckert RA, Elankumaran S, Milani A, et al. Detection of a new Mycobacterium species in wild striped bass in the Chesapeake Bay. J Clin Microbiol 2001;39(2):710–5.

[23] Hughes KP, Duncan RB, Smith SA. Mass (mycobacterial granuloma) in the oral cavity of cultured summer flounder, *Paralichthys dentatus*. Lab Anim (NY) 2002;31(3):25–7.

[24] Hughes KP, Smith SA. Clinical presentations of *Mycobacterium* sp. in summer flounder (*Paralichthys dentatus*) held in recirculating aquaculture systems. Virginia J Sci 2002;53(2):58.

[25] Chinabut S. Mycobacteriosis and norcardiosis. In: Woo PTK, Bruno DW, editors. Fish diseases and disorders. Volume 3: viral, bacterial, and fungal infections. New York: CAB International; 1999. p. 319–40.

[26] Adams A, Thompson KD, Morris D, et al. Development and use of monoclonal antibody probes for immunohistochemistry, ELISA and IFAT to detect bacterial and parasitic fish pathogens. Fish Shellfish Immunol 1995;5:537–47.

[27] Adams A, Thompson KD, McEwan H, et al. Development of monoclonal antibodies to *Mycobacterium spp.* isolated from Chevron Snakeheads and Siamese Fighting fish. J Aquat Anim Health 1996;8:208–15.

[28] Noga EJ. Fish disease diagnosis and treatment. Ames (IA): Iowa State University Press; 2000. p. 156–8.

[29] Conroy G, Conroy DA. Acid-fast bacterial infection and control in guppies (*Lebistes reticularis*) reared on an ornamental fish farm in Venezuela. Vet Rec 1999;144(7):177–8.

[30] Pasnik DJ, Vemulapalli R, Smith SA, et al. A recombinant vaccine expressing a mammalian Mycobacterium sp. antigen is immunostimulatory but not protective in striped bass. Vet Immunol Immunopathol 2003;95(1–2):43–52.

[31] Pasnik DJ, Smith SA. Development of a DNA vaccine for piscine mycobacteriosis. GAA (Global Aquaculture Alliance) Advocate 2003;6:24–5.

[32] Prouty MG, Correa NE, Barker LP, et al. Zebrafish *Mycobacterium marinum* model for mycobacterial pathogenesis. FEMS Microbiol Lett 2003;225(2):177–82.

[33] Noga EJ. Fish disease diagnosis and treatment. Ames (IA): Iowa State University Press; 2000. p. 208–11.

[34] Duszynski DW, Upton SJ, Couch L. The coccidia of the world. NSF-PEET and DEB 9521687-related resources. National Science Foundation and Partnership for Enhancing Expertise in Taxonomy (PEET). February 2004. http://biology.unm.edu/biology/coccidia/home.html.

[35] Upton SJ, Bristol JR, Gardner SL, et al. *Eimeria halleri* sp. n. (Apicomplexa: *Eimeriidae*) from the round stingray, *Urolophus halleri* (Rajiformes: *Dasyatidae*). Proc Helminthol Soc Wash 1986;53:110–2.

[36] Upton SJ, Duszynski DW. Development of Eimeria funduli in *Fundulus heteroclitus*. J Protozool 1982;29:66–71.

[37] Upton SJ, Gardner SL, Duszynski DW. The round stingray, *Urolophus halleri* (Rajiformes: Dasyatidae), as a host for *Eimeria chollaensis* sp. nov. (Apicomplexa: Eimeriidae). Can J Zool 1988;66:2049–52.

[38] Upton SJ, Stamper MA, Osborn AL, et al. A new species of *Eimeria* (Apicomplexa, Eimeriidae) from the weedy sea dragon *Phyllopteryx taeniolatus* (Osteichthyes: Syngnathidae). Dis Aquat Organ 2000;43(1):55–9.

[39] Borucinska JD, Frasca S Jr. Naturally occurring lesions and micro-organisms in two species of free-living sharks: the spiny dogfish, *Squalus acanthias* L., and the smooth dogfish, *Mustelus canis* (Mitchill), from the north-western Atlantic. J Fish Dis 2002;25(5):287.

[40] Stamper MA, Lewbart G, Barrington P, et al. *Eimeria southwelli* infection associated with high mortality of cownose rays. J Aquat Anim Health 1998;10:264–70.

[41] Stamper MA, Lewbart G, Barrington P, et al. Coccidial infections in cownose rays. Abstract from the 27th annual conference of the International Association for Aquatic Animal Medicine, Tennassee Aquarium, 11–15 May 1996. p. 29.

[42] Stamper MA, Lewbart G, Barrington P, et al. *Eimeria southwelli* infection associated with high mortality of cownose rays. J Aquat Anim Health 1998;10:264–70.

[43] Plumb JA. *Edwardsiella septicaemia*. In: Ingliss VR, Roberts J, Bromage NR, editors. Bacterial diseases of fishes. London: Blackwell Scientific Publications; 1993. p. 61–79.

[44] Goodwin AE, Lochman RT, Tieman DM, et al. Massive hepatic necrosis and nodular regeneration in largemouth bass fed diets high in available carbohydrate. J World Aquacult Soc 2002;33:466–77.

[45] Tidwell JH, Copyle SD, Woods TA. Species profile largemouth bass. SRAC Publication Number 722. Stoneville (MS): Southern Regional Aquaculture Center; 2000.

[46] Woo PTK. On cryptobiosis and infections by *Cryptobia*. J Fish Dis 2004;27(8):493.

[47] Mo TA, Poppe TT, Iversen L. Systemic hexamitosis in salt-water reared Atlantic salmon (*Salmo salar L.*). Bull Eur Assoc Fish Pathol 1990;10:69–70.

[48] Poppe TT, Mo TA, Iversen L. Disseminated hexamitosis in sea-caged Atlantic salmon *Salmo salar*. Dis Aquat Organ 1992;14:91–7.

[49] Floyd RF, Yanong R. *Cryptobia iubilans* in cichlids. Document VM104, Veterinary Medicine-Pathobiology Department, Florida Cooperative Extension Service, Institute of Food and Agricultural Sciences, University of Florida. Revised April 12, 2002. Visit the EDIS Web Site at http://edis.ifas.ufl.edu.

[50] Sterud E. Electron microscopical identification of the flagellate *Spironucleus torosa* (Hexamitidae) from burbot *Lota lota* (gadidae) with comments upon its probable introduction to this freshwater host. J Parasitol 1998;84:947–53.

[51] Sterud E, Mo TA, Poppe TT. Ultrastructure of *Spironucleus barkhanus* N. Sp. (Diplomonadida: Hexamitidae) from grayling *Thymallus thymallus* (L.) (Salmonidae) and Atlantic salmon Salmo salar L. (Salmonidae). J Eukaryot Microbiol 1997;44:399–407.

[52] Noga EJ. Fish disease diagnosis and treatment. Ames (IA): Iowa State University Press; 2000. p. 193–6.

[53] Turnbull J. Modified from 1998–1999 lecture notes for MSc course in Aquatic Veterinary Sciences and Aquatic Patho-biology. Institute of Aquaculture, University of Stirling, Stirling, Scotland.

[54] Noga EJ. Fish disease diagnosis and treatment. Ames (IA): Iowa State University Press; 2000. p. 55–250.

[55] Inglis V, Roberts Rj, Bromage NR. Bacterial diseases of fishes. Oxford, UK: Blackwell Scientific Publications; 1993.

[56] Hoffman GL. Parasites of North American freshwater fishes. Ithaca (NY): Comstock Publishing Associates; 1999.

[57] Lewbart GA. Self-assessment color review of ornamental fish. Ames (IA): Iowa State University Press; 1998.

[58] Woo PTK. Fish diseases and disorders. Volume 1: protozoan and metazoan infections. Oxford, UK: CABI Publishing; 1995.

[59] Leatherland JF, Woo PTK. Fish diseases and disorders. Volume 2: non-infectious disorders. Oxford, UK: CABI Publishing; 1999.

[60] Woo PTK, Bruno DW. Fish diseases and disorders. Volume 3: viral, bacterial, and fungal infections. Oxford, UK: CABI Publishing; 1999.

ELSEVIER
SAUNDERS

VETERINARY
CLINICS
Exotic Animal Practice

Vet Clin Exot Anim 8 (2005) 277–298

Clinical Reptile Gastroenterology

Mark A. Mitchell, DVM, MS, PhD*,
Orlando Diaz-Figueroa, DVM

*Department of Veterinary Clinical Sciences, Louisiana State University School of
Veterinary Medicine, Skip Bertman Drive, Baton Rouge, LA 70803, USA*

Reptiles have been successful in adapting to environmental niches, and survive in the face of competition from higher vertebrates, such as birds and mammals. This evolution has led to differences in the anatomy and physiology of different organ systems both between and within different orders of reptiles. Of all the different systems, the greatest diversity may be in the gastrointestinal tract. This variability in the anatomy and physiology of the reptilian gastrointestinal tract can pose a special problem for veterinarians when trying to make recommendations about nutrition, interpret diagnostic tests, and design a treatment regimen. The purpose of this article is to provide a review of the anatomy and physiology of the reptilian gastrointestinal tract. In addition, a review of diagnostic tests and common diseases associated with the gastrointestinal tract will be covered.

Anatomy and physiology

The reptilian gastrointestinal tract follows a similar pattern to that found in higher vertebrates, and includes the mouth, buccal cavity, oropharynx, esophagus, stomach, small intestine, large intestine, and colon. The terminus of the reptile gastrointestinal tract, the cloacae, is similar to that found in birds.

The oral cavity of the reptile is lined by mucous epithelium [1]. In squamates, the oral cavity has skin folds that seal the oral cavity; however, these structures are absent in crocodilians and chelonians. Reptile mucous membranes are generally a pale pink color. The mucous membranes should be moist. A thick ropey discharge is indicative of dehydration. Most snakes, chelonians, and lizards also have an opening in the hard palate that is

---

* Corresponding author.
E-mail address: mitchell@vetmed.lsu.edu (M.A. Mitchell).

1094-9194/05/$ - see front matter © 2005 Elsevier Inc. All rights reserved.
doi:10.1016/j.cvex.2005.01.008
vetexotic.theclinics.com

consistent with the choanae of birds. This passage allows reptiles to be breathe with their mouth closed. This passage should be evaluated for an obstruction (eg, foreign body, abscess, neoplasia) if a reptile is presented for open-mouthed breathing.

There is a high degree of variability in the different types of teeth and the location of the teeth in the oral cavity of reptiles. Crocodilians are thecodonts, and their teeth are only found lining the jaws. Lizards are generally classified as acrodonts or pleurodonts. Acrodontic teeth are located on the biting edge of the jaw and attach directly to the bone. Acrodontic teeth are not replaced when lost. Pleurodontic teeth are located in a groove in the jaw, and are generally replaced throughout the animal's life. Snakes have the most teeth of any reptile. In snakes, teeth are generally located on the dentary bones of the lower jaw and the premaxillae, maxillae, palatine, or pterygoid bones of the upper jaw. Venomous snakes and the helodermatid lizards have modifications to their teeth (fangs) to facilitate the delivery of venom.

Reptile saliva is produced by different salivary glands, including lingual, sublingual, palatine, and dental salivary glands. The labial glands of certain species of snakes and helodermatid lizards have been modified into venom glands. Reptile saliva appears to produce minimal proteolytic activity [2]. The multicellular mucous glands lining the oral cavity of squamates are well developed, while these glands are poorly developed in chelonians and crocodilians [2]. The mucous produced by these glands lubricates food and facilitates passage.

There is a high degree of variation in the shape, size, and function of reptile tongues between and within the different reptile orders. The snake tongue is a thin and protrusible, and has lost its mechanical capabilities in the interest of chemosensory specialization. Snakes tongues are heavily keratinized, and have relatively few taste buds [3]. Lizard tongues are generally mobile and protrusible, and generally have numerous taste buds [4]. In these animals, the tongue serves both chemosensory and mechanical functions. Certain lizards, such as varanids and lacertids, also have heavily keratinized tongues and relatively few taste buds, and are more similar to snake tongues [3]. Chelonians generally have fleshy tongues that have numerous taste buds. The Jacobson's organ, or vomeronasal organ, is a chemosensory structure found in squamates and chelonians, but is absent in crocodilians [5]. When present, it assists in the interpretation of chemical scents.

The reptile glottis is located on the floor of the oral cavity at the base of the tongue. The glottis is surrounded by two arytenoid cartilages and one cricoid cartilage. Crocodilians and chelonians have complete tracheal rings, while the squamates have incomplete tracheal rings. The snake glottis is highly moveable, which enables them to breathe while ingesting large meals.

The openings to the eustacian tubes are located in the dorsal/dorsolateral pharynx. The eustacian tubes connect the oral cavity to the middle ear and regulate pressure within the ear. Aural abscesses are a common problem encountered in captive and wild chelonians, and may be associated with ascending infections from the oral cavity. Snakes do not have eustacian tubes or a middle ear.

The reptile esophagus serves several important functions, including transporting ingesta to the stomach, serving as a temporary storage for food, and aiding in both mechanical and enzymatic digestion. Sea turtles and some species of tortoise use the strong muscles of the esophagus to crush food and initiate mechanical digestion [6]. Enzymatic digestion may occur in the distal esophagus from gastric reflux or the production of pepsin [6]. The anatomic and physiologic features of the reptile esophagus are fairly consistent between orders, with few exceptions. However, the length and proportion of the gastrointestinal tract represented by the esophagus can vary significantly. This is especially evident in snakes, which have a longer esophagus compared with chelonians, crocodilians, and lizards. The lining of the proximal esophagus is generally characterized by longitudinal folds, while the distal esophagus has broad and flat folds [7]. The width of these folds can be highly variable between species. Sea turtles have unique conical and cornified papillae lining the esophagus. The esophagus is lined with ciliated cells and goblet cells, and the distribution of these cells can vary within the esophagus. The muscularis mucosae is generally located in the caudal esophagus, but may be absent in chelonians. The tunica muscularis is comprised of both circular and longitudinal smooth muscle.

Reptile stomachs are comprised of fundic (corpus) and pars pylorica regions. The pars pylorica can be grossly distinct or subtle in appearance. Some species of chelonians, crocodilians, and lizards have a prominent cardiac region. In crocodilians, the corpus is comprised of thick muscle, and is analogous to the gizzard of birds. Rugae may be prominent within the stomach or absent. The gastric mucosa of the reptilian stomach produces a variety of enzymes, hydrochloric acid, and pepsin.

The primary functions of the reptile stomach are to store and digest food. The highly distensible nature of the reptilian stomach enables these animals to store large meals. Digestion of food occurs both via enzymatic and mechanical processes. The rate of digestion for reptiles may vary depending on body temperature, hydration status, food type, and meal size, and the general health of the reptile. Blain and Campbell [8] reported that a boa constrictor (*Constrictor constrictor*) required 120 hours to digest a rodent skeleton. However, it was difficult to interpret these results as the environmental temperature that the animal was maintained under was not reported. When temperature is optimized, the digestive rate is .25 to .33 the time required at an inappropriate environmental temperature [6]. Venom can also increase the rate of digestion. The venomous Jararacussu snake (*Bothrops jararacussu*) can digest a rodent prey in approximately 4 to 5 days if the prey is injected with venom, while it may take as much as 12 to 14 days without the venom [9]. The digestion of food occurs as a result of both enzymatic processes and the production of hydrochloric acid. Pepsinogen digests proteins, and is regulated by both temperature and gastric pH. The production and action of pepsinogen is dramatically increased in a strongly acidic environment and when the reptile is maintained at an optimal environmental temperature. Gastric pH is also affected by core body temperature. Another factor that can affect the gastric pH of a reptile is whether the animal had a recent meal. The gastric pH of anorectic reptiles can be >3.0. Optimal gastric pH ranges for reptiles are likely between 2.0 to 2.5 [10,11]. Because the secretion of hydrochloric acid, enzymes, and pepsinogen are temperature related, veterinarians should stress the importance of maintaining these animals at an optimal temperature. Failure to provide an appropriate environmental temperature could lead to decreased gastrointestinal motility and digestion, and the putrefaction of digesta.

The intestine continues the process of digesting food products, and is also the primary site for the absorption of nutrients. The length of the reptilian intestine varies with the type of diet the animal consumes. In general, the herbivore intestine is longer than the omnivore or carnivore intestine, while the omnivore intestine is longer than the carnivore intestine. Herbivorous lizards also tend to be larger in size than their carnivorous counterparts. This physical difference has been attributed to several potential theories, including that large quantities of plant material are more readily accessible than small packets of energy (insects), that large carnivores that compete with mammals are unsuccessful, and that the large size of the herbivore coupled with a greater thermal inertia reduces the amount of energy required to expend to thermoregulation [6]. Longitudinal folds within the reptilian intestine allow for an increased surface area for absorption, and also enable the intestine to distend and accommodate large quantities of digesta. A range of enzymes and bile salts, similar to mammals, is produced by the pancreas and liver. The pH (6.5–8.0) of the reptile intestine may vary, ranging from slightly acidic to slightly alkaline.

There is generally a gross distinction between the small intestine and colon in herbivorous reptiles; however, this difference may not be as evident in carnivorous reptiles. In herbivorous chelonians and lizards, the colon serves as a site for postgastric fermentation. Diet is not the only predictor of the presence and size of a colon, as a *Calotes jubatus*, an insectivore, and *Tupinambus teguixinm*, an omnivore, both have proportionally larger caecae than some herbivorous lizards [12].

Gastrointestinal motility can be affected by a number of different extrinsic and intrinsic factors [6]. In fasted reptiles, gastric motility is characterized by two phases: single short duration contractions, and longer contractions dispersed over a greater duration. Gastric tone is generally unchanged during a fast. Once the reptile has ingested a meal, the contractions increase. The rate that food passes through the gastrointestinal tract can vary with the volume, type and composition of the food, environmental and core body temperature, type and length of the gastrointestinal tract, and health of the reptile [6]. In small carnivorous squamates, food may pass through the gastrointestinal tract in as few as 2 to 4 days, while in large snakes, and herbivorous chelonians and lizards, it may require 3 to 5 weeks.

The cloaca and vent represent the terminus of the gastrointestinal tract. The cloaca is comprised of the urodeum, coprodeum, and proctodeum. The urodeum is the site of attachment for the urinary bladder, ureters, and reproductive tract. The coprodeum is the terminus of the colon. Both the coprodeum and urodeum empty into the proctodeum. Although the cloaca is routinely considered nothing more than the terminus of the gastrointestinal, reproductive, and excretory systems, it also plays an important role in the active absorption of electrolytes and the passive absorption of fluids.

There reptilian gall bladder and pancreas play important roles in the digestion and processing of nutrients. In chelonians, crocodilians, and most lizards, the gallbladder is contiguous with the liver. In some lizards, and most snakes, the gallbladder is located some distance from the liver, and conveys bile from the liver to the duodenum via a thin-walled cystic duct. In chelonians, the pancreatic and bile ducts enter the pylorus instead of the duodenum. Bile is stored in the gall bladder, and plays important roles in the digestion, absorption, and excretion of fat [13]. Triglycerides are digested by a mixture of lipases and bile into a solution of bile salts, monoglycerides, and fatty acids. The small molecular size of these products enables them to be absorbed via the enterocytes. Bile may also contain small concentrations of enzymes, such as amylase.

The function of the reptilian pancreas is similar to the mammalian pancreas. In chelonians and lizards, the pancreas is closely associated with the stomach and duodenum. The snake pancreas is located caudal to the stomach, and is generally found near the gallbladder and spleen. In some snakes, the pancreatic and splenic tissues are intermixed and form a splenopancreas. The reptilian pancreas is comprised of both exocrine and endocrine tissues. The exocrine tissues secrete digestive enzymes, including amylolytic, proteolytic, and lipolytic enzymes. Chitinase is also produced in the pancreas in those species that feed on prey that use chitin in their exoskeleton. In addition to the enzymes, the pancreas secretes alkaline fluid to counter the low pH of the gastric juices. The functions of the enzymes produced by the pancreas are highly dependent on temperature and pH (>6.0). Amylolytic enzymes, such as amylase, are believed to be excreted in higher concentration in herbivores compared with carnivores. Chymotrypsin, trypsin, carboxypeptidase, and elastase are proteolytic enzymes that have been identified in reptiles [6]. The production of enzymes by the pancreas is tied to the feeding strategy of the reptile. Certain enzymes, such a chitinase and amylase, are produced in much higher concentrations in one reptile compared with another depending on the reptile's feeding strategy.

Gastrointestinal tract disease: diagnostic testing

Anamnesis and physical examination

Because many of the problems that reptiles are presented to the veterinarian for are directly related to inappropriate husbandry, it is important to collect a detailed anamnesis. For example, identifying possible deficiencies in the management of the reptile, such as chronic hypothermia, an inappropriate diet, or never having evaluated a wild-caught animal for parasites, may be used to determine potential etiologies for anorexia, and guide in the diagnosis of a case. Historic questions should be directed at developing an understanding of the owner's experience with reptiles, the reptile's environment and diet, the problem that the animal is being presented for, and the duration of the problem. Specific questions that may be asked include the environmental temperature range and humidity, enclosure size, substrate, lighting and photoperiod, enclosure furniture, sanitation protocol, animal density, exposure to commercial products (toxins), diet, frequency of feeding, water source, fecal and urine consistency and frequency, and disinfection protocol.

The physical examination should be thorough and complete. The nares and eyes should be clear and free of discharge. The ears, when present, should be examined for abnormal swelling, discharge, or ectoparasites. The conjunctiva should appear moist, and the eyes not sunken. The oral cavity should be examined for injuries, abscesses, granulomas, and hemorrhage. The mucous membranes should be pale pink and moist. The capillary refill time should be less than 1.5 seconds. The tongue should be moist and pale pink to pink in color. In snakes, varanids, and chameleons, the tongue sheath should be free of discharge and edema.The tongue should also be evaluated for normal function. Any damage to the snake or chameleon tongue can lead to anorexia. The teeth should be examined closely, and any missing teeth recorded in the animal's record. The entire skull should be palpated for any abnormal swellings. The integument should be evaluated for the presence of ectoparasites, thermal injuries, trauma, and dermatitis. The cervical region and organ systems within the coelomic cavity should be palpated for abnormalities. Although the palpation of the chelonian coelomic cavity is limited by the shell, abnormal findings may be identified via palpation through the axillary or inguinal fossae. Because snake anatomy is consistent across families, these animals lend themselves well to palpation. It is also important to perform a cardiac examination on a reptile during a routine physical examination. A damp paper towel can be placed over the skin in the area of the heart to reduce the potential for friction between the scales and bell housing, and increase the auditory sound. An ECG or crystal ultrasonic doppler can also be used to evaluate the heart.

Diagnostic testing

Although the anamnesis and physical examination can provide significant insight into the problems occurring in a reptile patient, a thorough
diagnostic plan will need to formulated to confirm a diagnosis. When
evaluating gastrointestinal disease in a reptile, it is generally best to perform
the diagnostic assays in a series. An initial screen may include a complete
blood count, plasma biochemistries, microbiologic testing, fecal examination, and survey radiographs. Once these results have been collected and
interpreted, a second tier of diagnostics may be done, including a contrast
radiographic exam, ultrasound, toxicologic/infectious disease testing,
endoscopy, or surgical exploration. A third tier of diagnostics to consider,
when it is economically feasible, may include magnetic resonance imaging
(MRI) or CT scans.

The first tier of diagnostic tests can provide important information
regarding the physiologic status of the patient, and are relatively inexpensive
and noninvasive. Reptiles with gastrointestinal disease routinely have an
inflammatory leukogram. The elevated white counts are generally associated
with a heterophilia and a monocytosis. Anemia is also a frequent finding in
chronic inflammatory diseases associated with the gastrointestinal tract.
Alterations in the enzymes, electrolytes, and proteins are not uncommon in
reptiles with gastrointestinal disease. Reptiles with a history of regurgitation
or diarrhea may develop alterations in their sodium, potassium, and
chloride levels. The results of the electrolytes should also be evaluated in
light of dehydration, as they can become falsely elevated in dehydrated
reptiles. Aspartate aminotransferase (AST) and creatine kinase (CK) are
frequently elevated when there is damage to the smooth muscle of the
intestine or skeletal muscle catabolism as a result of long-term cachexia.
AST can also become elevated with liver disease, and elevations in the AST
without an elevated CK may be indicative of hepatitis. Historically,
veterinarians classified the majority of the problems encountered in reptile
medicine as bacterial infections. The primary reason for this was because
of the tendency of veterinarians to submit cultures as part of a routine
screening. Veterinarians should use caution when interpreting these results,
as it is not uncommon to isolate organisms that are a component of the
indigenous flora. In most cases, when a bacterial organism is a pathogen,
a heavy growth of the organism will be isolated on the culture plate, and the
animal will have clinical signs associated with an infection. Be sure to
discuss these cultures with your laboratory to prevent the unnecessary use of
antibiotics. Fecal material should be collected and submitted for a parasi-
tologic examination. The examination should include both a direct saline
smear and fecal flotation. If encysted protozoa are suspected, than a smear
should also be made using Lugol's iodine stain. If *Cryptosporidium* spp is
suspected, than a sample should be submitted for an acid-fast stain or for
a commercial enzyme-linked immunosorbent assays (ELISA). Radiographs

can be used to rule out foreign material and abnormal masses within the gastrointestinal tract.

The second tier of diagnostics provides the opportunity to characterize a specific disease process or etiology. These assays are generally more expensive and invasive. Contrast radiography and ultrasound provide a more detailed review of the gastrointestinal tract. Because environmental temperature can affect gastric motility, it is important to maintain the reptile at an optimal temperature to ensure that the contrast will pass through the gastrointestinal tract at an appropriate rate. Contrasts series in reptiles, especially the herbivores, can take extended periods of time (20–30 days), so an extended series of films may have to be taken. Endoscopic examination and surgical exploration provide direct visualization of the gastrointestinal tract. Endoscopy is less invasive, and should be pursued first. Historically, there were very few reptilian diagnostic assays available to the veterinarian. Fortunately, with the advent of new serologic and molecular assays veterinarians can evaluate a reptile patient for a specific infectious disease.

The third tier of diagnostic assays are generally performed last because they are expensive and of limited availability to most practitioners. Advanced diagnostic imaging, such as CT and MRI, can provide valuable information regarding the specific lesions within an organ. As these diagnostics become more available, and the expense associated with them decreases, there value to veterinarians working with reptiles will increase.

Common gastrointestinal diseases

Noninfectious diseases

Toxins

Gastrointestinal toxicosis from the ingestion of external toxins is not a common finding in captive herpetoculture. Lead toxicosis has been reported in a common snapping turtle (*Chelydra serpentina*) that presented for anorexia, and was found to have fishing gear and lead weights in the gastrointestinal tract [14]. The toxicosis was confirmed by measuring blood lead levels in the turtle. A case of lead toxicosis has also been reported in a Greek tortoise (*Testudo graeca*) [15]. The tortoise was found to have neurologic symptoms associated with the ingestion of a lead shot. Chelation therapy was initiated (sodium calcium edentate, 35 mg/kg, intramuscularly, every 24 hours until resolution), and the animal improved. Lead toxicosis has also been identified in a group of captive alligators at an alligator ranch. The animals were offered a diet of wild prekilled nutria. The alligators were found to be neurologic and anorectic. Necropsies on recently dead animals revealed a lead toxicosis. The lead shot used to kill the nutria was found to be the source of the lead contamination. Currently, there are no reference values available for blood heavy metal levels in reptiles. In cases where a heavy metal toxicosis is suspected, it would be prudent to measure blood levels of the heavy metal in a healthy example of the same species.

It is not uncommon for some herpetoculturists to feed their captive insectivorous reptiles wild-caught insects. However, there is an inherent danger to this, as many invertebrates produce toxins. The common firefly, *Photinus* spp, produces steroidal pyrones (lucibufagans) that are highly toxic to bearded dragons and other species of lizards. Ingestion of a single firefly is often fatal. If your clients wish to feed wild-caught insects, they should obtain a book on entomology or talk with a local entomologist to ensure that they are not feeding their reptile potentially toxic insects.

Gastrointestinal foreign bodies

Many reptiles are nonselective in their feeding habits and will ingest substrate surrounding their food items [6]. In addition, pica or geophagy is also a common practice in terrestrial reptiles. Some speculate that these animals ingest these items, like birds, to create gastroliths that assist with the mechanical digestion of foods, although this has not been proven.

In captivity, these practices can lead to the development of gastrointestinal foreign bodies that require medicinal or surgical treatment (Fig. 1). The majority of the cases, in the authors' experience, are found in insectivorous lizards that ingest substrate along with their invertebrate prey, and chelonians, which are known to be geophagic. The "digestible" calcium carbonate sands are the primary culprit in the lizard cases. Leopard geckos and bearded dragons can ingest large quantities of these products over time, leading to gastric impaction. Many of the newer cricket water products that are comprised of a synthetic material can also lead to gastric foreign bodies in captive insectivorous reptiles (Fig. 2). The authors have observed two cases in bearded dragons where the animals ingested a dehydrated cube from the cricket product, only to have it reexpand and rupture their stomachs. These products should not be placed into the reptile's enclosure.

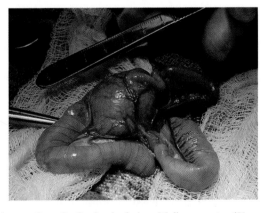

Fig. 1. Surgical correction of a foreign body in a Mali uromastyx (*Uromastyx maliensis*).

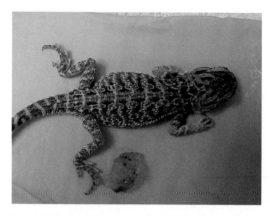

Fig. 2. This piece of synthetic gel used to water commercial feeder insects was removed from the stomach of this bearded dragon (*P vitticeps*).

Chelonians, especially omnivores and herbivores, are prone to ingest woody materials and rocks. In chelonians, these items generally gain passage through to the colon. Snakes are not prone to ingest inanimate objects; however; the authors have observed snakes to ingest coconut bark or aspen bedding while swallowing a prey item, and a large boa constrictor swallowed an electric heating pad that was inside the cage with the snake.

Reptiles with gastrointestinal foreign bodies may present with acute lethargy and anorexia. Regurgitation may be reported in the clinical history, especially in snakes. Snakes possess a poorly developed cardiac sphincter, thus permitting what can appear to be almost effortless regurgitation. Regurgitation is associated with pathology of the upper gastrointestinal tract, which includes the oral cavity, pharynx, esophagus, stomach, and small intestines. It is important to consider regurgitation as only a symptom of the underlying disease. Episodes of vomiting, as would be expected in dog or a cat, are very rare in reptiles. The history can also be much more chronic in nature, being characterized by gradual weight loss, lethargy, anorexia occurring over several months, and constipation. Melena, hematochezia, reduced fecal production, and pain associated with eating may also be reported.

With an acute onset of clinical signs, reptiles are usually lethargic, dehydrated, and depressed on physical examination. Reptiles with a chronic history will often be cachectic and dehydrated. Results of a complete blood count may reveal a decreased hematocrit (anemia), suggesting hemorrhage from the upper gastrointestinal tract; and a leukocytosis. Elevated hepatic and muscle enzymes, and electrolytes disturbances, may also occur with gastrointestinal foreign bodies.

Diagnostic images are an important diagnostic tool to pursue when evaluating a patient for a gastrointestinal foreign body. Metal and mineral foreign bodies can be detected using survey radiographs (Fig. 3). Rubber

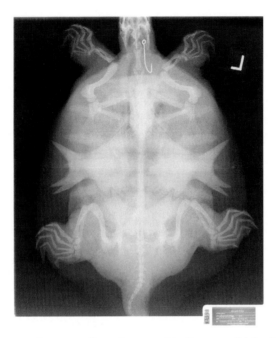

Fig. 3. This dorsoventral survey radiograph was used to diagnose a fish hook foreign body in this spiny soft-shelled turtle (*Apalone spinifera*).

and plastic materials may be more difficult to detect using survey radiographs. In these cases, a contrast series should be performed. Because the gastrointestinal motility of reptiles is longer than in mammals and birds, the contrast series may need to be extended over several days or weeks. Ultrasonography, CT, and MRI may be of a significant value in the diagnosis of the reptile in which evidence of a foreign body is questionable. Treatment generally requires surgical removal of the foreign body and recommendations to change the substrate to prevent reoccurrence.

Gastrointestinal neoplasia

Historically, neoplasia has not been considered a common finding in reptiles; however, as the captive husbandry programs improve and these animals live longer lives, veterinarians can expect to have more reptile neoplasia cases presented to their practice [1,16–21]. Neoplastic disorders should be considered in a differential diagnosis regardless of the age of the patient. Neoplastic diseases of the gastrointestinal system in reptiles may be a challenge to diagnose, even when a detailed diagnostic plan is followed.

Gastrointestinal neoplasia has been reported in all of the major reptilian orders [22]. Our current understanding behind the pathophysiology of reptile neoplasia is limited; however, recent research has identified viral and parasitic pathogens associated with the development of neoplasia in reptiles.

A C-type oncorna virus has been correlated to poikilotherm oncogenesis [20]. A recent case report of a hepatoma in an iguana (*Iguana iguana*) was found to be associated with viral-like inclusions in the neoplastic hepato-cytes [22]. Herpesvirus has recently been associated with the development of fibropapillomas in green sea turtle (*Chelonia mydas*). Although there are no confirmed case reports attributing parasite infestations to the induction of neoplasia in reptiles, there may be an association between a trematodes species and a papillomatous change observed in the gall bladder of a green sea turtle (*C mydas*) [23]. Future research to elucidate these relationships is needed.

The clinical signs attributed to gastrointestinal neoplasia in reptiles can vary, and may include emesis, hematoemesis, dysphagia, ptalyism, facial deformities, palpable masses, poor growth, anorexia, caudal coelomic distention, melena, minimal axial flexion of the posterior trunk, asymmetric cloacal enlargement, and constipation [1]. Hematology and plasma bio-chemistries can provide insight into the physiologic status of the reptile patient. Anemia, lymphopenia or lymphocytosis, heterophilia, and mono-cytosis may occur with cases of gastrointestinal neoplasia. Survey radio-graphs, contrast radiographs, and ultrasonography also may be used to support a diagnosis of gastrointestinal neoplasia. However, a final diagnosis can only be made from a fine needle aspirate and biopsy of the mass.

Our current understanding for the treatment of neoplasia in reptiles is limited. In general, treatment is dependent on the size, location, and type of neoplasm. Because of our limited experience with chemotherapy and radi-ation therapy in reptiles, surgical removal of the tumor is the most common treatment method. If surgical borders can be achieved, surgery is also con-sidered the preferred treatment.

Infectious diseases

Infectious diseases are the most common cause of gastrointestinal disease in captive reptiles. Many of the problems encountered with infectious diseases are the direct result of inappropriate husbandry and poor quarantine procedures. Many of the bacterial and fungal pathogens isolated from reptiles with gastrointestinal disease are a component of the indi-genous microflora. Under less than ideal environmental conditions, these opportunistic pathogens invade their host. Likewise, many of the parasites that reptiles harbor only become problematic when the host is on a poor diet and has a negative energy balance or is immunocompromised.

Viral diseases

The incidence of viral diseases in captive reptiles is increasing. This is most likely associated with improved diagnostics, and the emergence of new viral diseases resulting from the mixing of naïve species. Currently, the majority of the gastrointestinal disease cases attributed to viral diseases are limited to case reports. To confirm that a virus was responsible for a specific disease process, an experimental infection to fulfill Koch's postulate must be performed. Future research to elucidate the pathophysiology associated with these viruses is needed.

Herpes virus has become a significant pathogen in captive chelonians. The virus was first isolated from sea turtles in the 1970s, and has since been identified in other freshwater, marine, and terrestrial species of chelonians. Herpes virus transmission is likely spread via horizontal route. This virus can affect multiple organ systems, including the gastrointestinal, respiratory, argental, and central nervous systems. Clinical signs can vary, and may include rhinitis, conjunctivitis, necrotizing stomatitis, enteritis, pneumonia, and neurologic disease. A diagnosis of an active herpes viral infection can be made using viral culture, a reverse transcription polymerase chain reaction assay, or paired titers using a serum neutralization or ELISA assay. Affected animals should be provided appropriate supportive care (eg, fluids, enterals, and antibiotics) to control clinical signs. Acyclovir has been used with some success by reducing viral replication, but will not likely eradicate the virus. Affected animals should be culled from captive populations to reduce the likelihood of transmitting the disease to other animals.

Inclusion body disease (IBD) is a major disease in boids and pythons, and has been associated with significant mortalities. A retrovirus is suspected to be the etiologic agent of IBD, but this has not been confirmed. The exact mechanisms for the transmission of IBD are not known; however, it appears to be spread horizontally and possibly through contact with snake mites (*Ophionyssus natricis*). The disease presentations in boids and pythons can vary, but they are generally associated with the gastrointestinal and central nervous systems. Chronic regurgitation is one of the early signs associated with this disease. As the disease progresses, snakes develop neurologic signs, including the loss of their righting reflex, tremors, and disorientation. The severe neurologic signs are more frequently reported in the pythons, and the disease in these snakes' progresses faster than in boids. Snakes generally succumb to this disease as a result of secondary infections and starvation. Surgical biopsies of the pancreas, esophageal tonsils, or kidney may be used to make an antemortem diagnosis. The trademark histologic lesion associated with this disease is eosinophilic intracytoplasmic inclusions. Currently, there is no effective treatment for this virus. Affected animals should be culled from a population and euthanized to prevent the spread of the virus to other snakes.

Adenoviral infections in bearded dragons (*Pogona vitticeps*) have become problematic in many collections in recent years. Although this virus was first reported in Australia in the early 1980s, the virus did not become problematic in the United States until the mid 1990s. Since that time, this virus has spread through numerous bearded dragon populations in the

United States, and should be considered endemic. Transmission of the virus is presumed to be horizontal (fecal–oral). This virus is more problematic in juvenile dragons than in adult animals. The clinical signs associated with this virus may include anorexia, weight loss, limb paresis, diarrhea, and opisthotonous. Concurrent dependovirus and coccidial infections have also been observed in neonatal bearded dragons. Antemortem biopsies of the liver, stomach, esophagus, or kidney may be used to confirm an adenoviral diagnosis. The classic histologic lesions associated with this virus are basophilic intranuclear inclusion bodies. There is no effective treatment for adenoviral infections in bearded dragons, although success may be had with fluid therapy, enteral support, and antibiotics to prevent opportunistic bacteria infections. Because the epidemiology of this virus is not known, clients should be made aware of the importance of quarantine and screening.

Bacterial diseases

Historically, bacterial pathogens were blamed for the vast majority of all diseases reported in reptiles. The primary reason for this was related to our limited range of diagnostic tests. Bacterial cultures were routinely collected from reptiles at the time of examination and submitted, but few other assays were performed. Because the gastrointestinal flora of reptiles is active, it was unlikely that a bacterial organism would not be isolated. The problem occurred when veterinarians tried to interpret the results and determine if an isolate was a true pathogen or a commensal. Many of the commensal microbes of the reptile gastrointestinal flora are also opportunistic pathogens (eg, *Salmonella* spp, *Escherichia coli*, *Citrobacter* spp), so differentiating their status could be difficult. Discussing the growth of the organism with your laboratory could be beneficial, as heavy growth of a microbe in the face of an enteritis is supportive of a bacterial infection. Additional diagnostics, including hematology and biopsies of affected areas, can also be used in combination with culture to confirm a diagnosis.

Infectious stomatitis is a common finding in captive reptiles. It is important to realize that this term is a clinical sign, and not necessarily a diagnosis. Reptiles with infectious stomatitis may present with inflammation of the mucosa, abscesses, granulomas, or petechial hemorrhages. Historically, samples of these lesions were collected and submitted for culture. A number of different bacteria may be isolated from the oral cavity of affected reptiles, including *Salmonella* spp, *E coli*, *Pseudomonas* spp, *Aeromonas* spp, *Citrobacter* spp, *Pasteurella* spp, *Alcaligenes* spp, and *Klebsiella* spp Again, all of these organisms can be both commensal and pathogenic, so the interpretation of the results should be based on additional ancillary testing. Occasionally, an atypical microbe will be isolated from a lesion in the oral cavity, such as in two boa constrictor cases in which a *Mycobacteria* sp. and a *Mycobacterium chelonei* were isolated [24,25]. If it is determined that the bacterial isolate is associated with a stomatitis, then antibiotic sensitivity testing should be done to guide treatment.

Acute gastritis in reptiles has been associated with severe thermal burns, major surgery, anti-inflammatory agents, corticosteroid administration, toxins, and infectious diseases. Affected reptiles may present for anorexia, regurgitation, and melena. The symptoms usually abate after the causative agent has been removed. In contrast, chronic gastritis is more difficult to manage because of the pathologic changes that have occurred in the reptile, such as severe ulceration and granuloma formation. Chronic gastritis has been associated with chronic poor husbandry, neoplasia, and bacterial infections. Cases of diptheritic necrotizing gastritis has been reported in a rosy boa (*Lichanura trivirgata*) associated with *Salmonella arizonae* [26]. In addition, atrophic gastritis has been reported in Hermann's tortoises (*Testudo hermanni*) [27]. The disease is characterized by atrophy and inflammation of the glandular component of the gastric mucosa and loss of the oxynticopeptic cells with their subsequent replacement by mucus cells.

Enteritis is one of the most common presentations at the authors' practice. Gram-negative bacteria are the most common agent isolated in these cases. The most common isolates are similar to those that are isolated from the oral cavity, stomach, and cloaca, and include *E coli, Klebsiella* spp, *Salmonella* spp, *Enterococcus* spp, *Pseudomonas* spp, *Serratia* spp, *Proteus* spp, *Citrobacter* spp, *Alcaligines* spp, and *Pasteurella* spp Gram-positive bacteria also may be isolated from reptiles with enteritis. The most common Gram-positive organisms isolated from reptiles in the authors' practice include *Clostridium* spp, *Corynebacterium* spp, *Enterococcus* spp, *Streptococcus* spp, and *Staphylococcus* spp Acid-fast bacteria, such as *Mycobacteria* spp, may also be isolated from the gastrointestinal tract of reptiles, and should be considered when a reptile presents for a bacterial enteritis that is nonresponsive to antibiotics. The treatment for bacterial enteritis should include supportive care, with specific attention to the hydration status of the animal, an antibiotic based on sensitivity testing, and the optimization of the diet. It is important to provide adequate dietary fiber to encourage the growth of normal gastrointestinal flora when dealing with herbivorous reptiles. Transfaunating the intestine with indigenous microflora from a clinically normal reptile may be considered, but the true value of this procedure is unknown.

Fungal disease

Fungal-related gastrointestinal disease is rare in captive and free-ranging reptiles. The reason for the dirth of cases may, again, be attributed to the fact that clinicians are not testing for fungal agents. *Paecilomyces lilacinus* has been isolated from the oral cavity, gastric mucosa, and liver of an Aldabra tortoise (*Geochelone gigantean*) [28]. A *Geotrichum* sp was isolated from a cloacal lavage of a Honduran milk snake (*Lampropeltis triangulum hondurensis*) with mucous colitis, and mucormycosis (*Rhizopus* spp) was diagnosed in a diamond python (*Morelia spilota spilota*) with clinical signs of hematochezia [29]. An *Aspergillus* sp has also been isolated from a periodontal osteomyelitis in a panther chameleon (*Furcifer pardalis*) [30].

The diagnosis of a fungal disease should be based on a series of diagnostic tests, including blood work, diagnostic imaging techniques, fungal culture, and histopathology. Histopathologic examination of impression smears, biopsies, or necropsy specimens are required to identify and characterize the morphologic characteristics of the fungal elements. Characteristics such as the width of hyphae, presence or absence of septae, type and size of reproductive structures, colony morphology, and optimum incubation temperature are used to identify and classify fungi. Culture may require some specialization, and laboratories should be contacted to obtain instructions for specific sampling techniques to minimize bacterial overgrowth of cultures. Successful treatment of fungal infections generally requires surgical debridement of an affected site, topical or systemic antifungal agents, and supportive care. Treatment can be prolonged.

Parasitic disease

Protozoa are a common finding on routine fecal examinations. The majority of the gastrointestinal protozoal species characterized from reptiles are nonpathogenic. Protozoal populations are influenced by a variety of factors within the gastrointestinal tract, including pH, organism density, substrate availability, and interprotozoal predation. The protozoal flora can also have an affect on the bacterial flora due to substrate competition and predation. Many veterinarians are unsure of whether they should treat the protozoal organisms they find on routine screens. However, treatment should only be pursued if there are clinical signs consistent with a protozoal enteritis.

Coccidia are obligate pathogens in reptiles, and are generally host specific. Lizards have the most distinct coccidian species, followed by snakes [31]. There have been eight species of *Eimeria* and two of species of *Isospora* reported in crocodilians [32]. Coccidia are transmitted via the fecal–oral route. The pathologic changes that have been associated with these parasites, include sloughing of the intestinal lining, hyperplasia of the epithelium and enterocytes, and the movement of inflammatory cells into the mucosa [31].

Isospora amphiboluri is the coccidian parasite of bearded dragons, and this parasite is endemic in the captive dragons in the United States. Like many of the reptile pathogens introduced into the United States, it has been well disseminated because of a lack of any effective quarantine system in herpetoculture. This parasite can cause significant morbidity and moderate mortalities in juvenile bearded dragons. Adult dragons are generally asymptomatic. Affected dragons may be anorectic, and have weight loss and diarrhea. Eventually, the juvenile dragons become extremely dehydrated if they are not provided supportive fluid therapy. This parasite can be difficult to eradicate. The authors find that sulfadimethoxine (50 mg/kg, orally, once a day for 21–28 days) and Trimethoprim sulfadiazine (30 mg/kg, orally, once; followed by 15 mg/kg orally once a day for 21–28 days) produce the best results and can reduce shedding in infected dragons.

Cryptosporidiosis is a major concern in herpetoculture. Although cryptosporidiosis is associated with high morbidity in mammals, it is generally self-limiting. In reptiles, this parasite is not apparently self-limiting, and is associated with high mortalities. Historically, there was one described species in reptiles (*Cryptosporidium serpentis*). More recently, a species has been described in lizards (*Cryptosporidium saurophilum*) [33]. Although no species has been speciated from chelonians, there is one report of cryptosporidiosis in a green sea turtle (*Chelonia mydas*) [34]. Cryptosporidiosis is transmitted via the fecal–oral route. The clinical signs most frequently reported in snakes include chronic regurgitation, weight loss, and hypertrophic gastritis. In snakes, the parasites infect the mucin-secreting cells of the stomach, and their life cycle is hastened by the ingestion of food. The life cycle in lizards appears to be different, as *C saurophilum* primarily infects the intestines, rather than the stomach [33]. Cryptosporidial diagnosis can be achieved by submitting feces (Fig. 4) or stomach contents for an acid-fast stain, a commercial ELISA used to diagnose *Cryptosporidium parvum* and *Giardia* sp in humans, or a polymerase chain reaction assay. Because these parasites may be shed transiently, it is important to submit

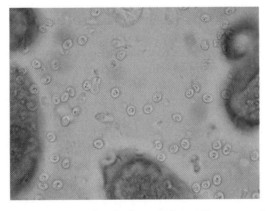

Fig. 4. Numerous *C serpentis* oocysts in a fecal sample from a Texas rat snake (*Elaphe obsoleta lindheimeri*).

serial samples for testing. In snakes, a biopsy of the stomach can also be diagnostic.

There is currently no consistently effective treatment for cryptosporidiosis in reptiles, and the organisms are also resistant to many disinfectants. There has been one study published that found that bovine hyperimmune colostrum could be used to eliminate *C saurophilum* from savannah monitors [35]. In the same study, the colostrum had no affect on *C saurophilum* in leopard geckos. Preventing the introduction of this parasite to reptile collections should be considered a priority. The authors recommend that reptiles be quarantined for a minimum of 90 days and five fecal samples submitted for testing. Infected animals should be culled from a collection.

Trematodes are a fairly common finding in wild-caught reptiles. The majority of the trematodes affecting reptiles are digenetic, and the reptile may serve as an intermediate host or as a definitive host. Veterinarians are more likely to encounter those trematodes in which the reptile serves as the definitive host, as eggs may be shed in the sputum or feces. Fortunately, these parasites are self-limiting in captivity because they require a gastropod intermediate host. When reptiles serve as an intermediate host, the trematodes are often encysted in tissues and pose minimal problems. Most of these infestations are diagnosed on necropsy. *Ochetosoma* spp, *Stomatotrema* spp, and *Pneumatophilus* spp are flukes that are routinely found in the oral cavity of ophidians, while *Odhneriotrema* spp is the most common fluke in alligators [36]. Trematodes of aquatic turtles are frequently found in the alimentary tract, liver, gallbladder, urinary bladder, and circulatory system; however, clinical disease associated with these infestations is rare [36]. Praziquantel (5–8 mg/kg, orally or subcutaneously, every 10–14 days) is considered the treatment of choice for trematodes; however, this recommendation was based on anecdotal findings.

Proteocephalidae, Pseudophyllidae, and Mesocestoididae represent the cestode families important in clinical reptile medicine. These cestodes have an indirect life cycle. The adults are located in the lumen, and shed proglottids with the feces. These parasites do not generally cause clinical disease, unless the there is a high density of parasites. In lizards and snakes, proteocephalid cestodes are the most common tapeworm. *Ophiotaenia* spp (snakes), *Proteocephalus* spp (lizards), and *Crepidoboyhrium* spp (boids), have been found to induce intestinal necrosis, epithelial loss, and round cell infiltrate within the tunica muscularis [37,38]. Members of the order Pseudophyllidae have also been isolated from snakes and lizards. The most common pathologic findings associated with these cestodes are ulcers in intestinal mucosa, hemorrhage, and edema. Praziquantel is also frequently used to eradicate cestodes, and the recommended dose is similar to that used for trematodes.

Nematodes are a common finding in a reptile fecal examination. Adult nematodes found within the gastrointestinal tract are generally considered to be parasitic, while free-living forms are generally not. Both wild-caught and captive-bred reptiles may present with nematodiasis. A lack of effective quarantine programs, and the regular mixing of wild-caught and captive-bred reptiles in collections, has led to the widespread dissemination of these parasites.

Oxyurids, or pinworms, are the most common nematodes encountered in the authors' practice. These nematodes are generally considered to be nonpathogenic in reptiles; however, high densities of these worms can lead to abnormal gastromotility, impaction, and possibly intussusception (Fig. 5). The oxyurids are primarily found in the lower intestine and colon, and are thought to play an important role in the digestion of food herbivorous reptiles. The life cycle of oxyurids is direct, and these the eggs are spread via the oral fecal route.

Strongyloid nematodes can be found throughout the alimentary tract (Fig. 6). Three genera of strongyles, including *Diaphanocephaloidea* spp, *Oswaldocruzia* spp, and *Kalicephalus* spp, have been found to infest lizards and snakes. These parasites can cause severe hemorrhagic ulceration, perforation, and gastrointestinal obstruction [39,40]. *Capillaria* spp, is the only known trichurid to infest squamates and crocodilians. These nematodes primarily infest the intestine, but have been found in other organs such as the liver and gonads. This parasite also has a direct life cycle.

Anisakidae and Ascarididae are the two most common families of ascarids to infest reptiles [39]. From the family Ascarididae, three species has been shown to parasitize snakes. *Ophidascaris labiatopapillosa* has been reported in North American snakes after ingestion of frogs and rodents, which serve as intermediate hosts [39]. *Ophidascaris moreliae* and *Polydelphis anoura*, have been found to infect pythons, especially if the larva are released into the water [41]. Two genera have also been found to affect crocodilians: *Dujardinascaris* and *Paratrichosoma*. High densities of these ascarids can cause gastrointestinal perforation and ulceration [39].

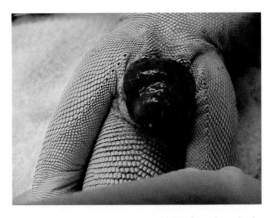

Fig. 5. Cloacal prolapse in a green iguana resulting from intestinal nematodiasis.

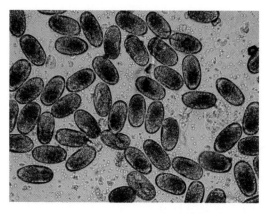

Fig. 6. This fecal float from a Texas rat snake revealed a large number of *Strongyle* eggs.

There are several different antiparasitics that may be used to manage nematode infestations. Fenbendazole may be used at 25 to 50 mg/kg by mouth once a day for 5 days and repeated in 10 days, ivermectin at 0.2 mg/kg intramuscularly every 2 weeks for a minimum of two treatments, or albendazole at 50 mg/kg once. Chelonians should not be treated with ivermectin as it is potentially neurotoxic.

Summary

Gastroenterology represents an important specialty within clinical reptile medicine. Veterinarians should become familiar with the unique anatomic and physiologic differences between reptiles to improve their management of these cases. In addition, veterinarians should use available diagnostic tests to confirm the presence of gastrointestinal disease. With the current advancements in reptile medicine, there is no reason these cases cannot be pursued to their fullest.

References

[1] Benson KG. Reptilian gastrointestinal diseases. Sem Avin Exot Pet Med 1998;8:90–7.
[2] Kochva E. Phylogeny of oral glands in reptiles as related to the origin and evolution of snakes. In: Rosenberg P, editor. Toxins: animal, plant and microbial. Oxford: Pergamon Press; 1978. p. 29–37.
[3] Young BA. On the absence of taste buds in monitor lizards (*Varanus*) and snakes. J Herpetol 1997;31:130–7.
[4] Schwenk K. Occurrence, distribution and functional significance of taste buds in lizards. Copeia 1985;91–101.
[5] Parsons TS. The nose and Jacobson's organ. In: Gans C, Parsons TS, editors. Biology of the reptilia. Vol. 2: morphology. London: Academic Press; 1970. p. 99–191.

[6] Skoczylas R. Physiology of the digestive tract. In: Gans C, Gans KA, editors. Biology of the reptilia. Vol. 8: physiology. London: Academic Press; 1978. p. 589–717.

[7] Parsons TS, Cameron JE. Internal relief of the digestive tract. In: Gans C, Parsons TS, editors. Biology of the reptilia. Vol. 6: morphology E. London: Academic Press; 1977. p. 159–223.

[8] Blain AW, Campbell KN. A study of the digestive phenomena in snakes with the aid of a Roentgen ray. AJR Am J Roentgenol 1942;48:229–39.

[9] Reichert E. Bothrops jararacussu. Bl Aquar Kunde 1936;47:228–31.

[10] Vonk HJ. Die biologische bedeutung des pH-optimums der verdauunsenzyme bei den vertebraten. Ergebn Enzymol 1939;8:55–88.

[11] Diefenbach CO. Gastric function in Caiman crocodiles (Crocodilia: Reptilia) I. Rate of gastric digestion and gastric motility as a function of temperature. Comp Biochem Physiol 1975;51A:259–65.

[12] Lönnenberg E. On some points of relation between the morphological structure of the intestine and the diets of reptiles. Bih Svensk Vet Ak Handl 1902;28:1–51.

[13] Haslewood GAD. Bile salts evolution. J Lipid Res 1967;8:535–50.

[14] Borkowski R. Lead poisoning and intestinal perforation in a snapping turtle (*Chelydra serpentina*) due to fishing gear ingestion. J Zoo Wildl Med 1997;28:109–14.

[15] Chitty JR. Lead toxicosis in a Greek tortoise (*Testudo graeca*). Proc ARAV, Minneapolis, MN; 2003. p. 101.

[16] Latimer K, Rich GA. Colonic adenocarcinoma in a corn snake (*Elaphe guttata guttata*). J Zoo Wildl Med 1998;29:344–6.

[17] Leonardi L, Grazioli O, Mechelli L, et al. Gastric mucinous adenocarcinoma in a diamond python (*Morelia spilotes spilotes*). Proc ARAV, Reno, NV; 2002. p. 63.

[18] Funk R.S. Cloacal adenocarcinoma in three juvenile diamond pythons (*Morelia spilotes spilotes*). Proc ARAV, Reno, NV; 2000. p. 101–3.

[19] Fickbohm BL, Kennedy GA. Gastric adenocarcinoma in a carpet python (*Morelia spilotes variegata*). J Herp Med Surg 1999;9:28–9.

[20] Hardy WD, McClelland AJ. Oncogenic RNA viral infections. In: Steele JH, editor. CRC handbook series in zoonoses. Vol. II. Cleveland: CRC Press; 1981. p. 321–33.

[21] Schillinger L, Selleri P, Frye FL. Hepatoma in a green iguana (*Iguana iguana*), accompanied by viral-like inclusions. Proc ARAV, Reno, NV; 2002. p. 75.

[22] Martin JC, Schelling SH, Pokras MA. Gastric adenocarcinoma in a Florida indigo snake (*Drymarchon corais couperi*). J Zoo Wildl Med 1994;25:133–7.

[23] Smith GM, Coates C, Nigrelli R. A papillomatous disease of the gallbladder associated with infection by flukes occurring in the marine turtle (*Chelonia mydas*). Zoologica 1941;26:13.

[24] Olson GH, Hodgin C, Peckman R. Infectious stomatitis associated with *Mycobacterium* sp. in a boa constrictor. Comp Anim Pract 1987;8:47–9.

[25] Quesenberry KE, Jacobson ER, Allen JL, et al. Ulcerative stomatitis and subcutaneous granuloma caused by *Mycobacterium chelonei* in a boa constrictor. J Am Vet Med Assoc 1986;189:1131.

[26] Oros J, Rodriguez L, Herraez P, et al. Respiratory and digestive lesions caused by *Salmonella arizonae* in two snakes. J Comp Pathol 1996;115:185–9.

[27] Zwart P, van der Gaag I. Atrophic gastritis in a Hermann's tortoise (*Testudo hermanni*) and two red-eared sliders (*Chrysemys scripta elegans*). Am J Vet Res 1981;42:2191–5.

[28] Heard DJ, Cantor GH, Jacobson ER, et al. Hyalohyphomycosis caused by *Paecilomyces lilacinus* in an Aldabra tortoise. J Am Vet Med Assoc 1986;189:1143–5.

[29] Raiti P. Mycotic gastroenteritis in a diamond python (*Morelia spilota spilota*) and two Honduran milk snakes (*Lampropeltis triangulum hondurensis*). Proc ARAV, Orlando, FL; 1996. p. 97.

[30] Heatley JJ, Mitchell MA, Williams J, et al. Fungal periodontal osteomyelitis in a chameleon (Furcifer pardalis): J Herp Med Surg 2001;11:7–12.

[31] Greiner EC. Coccidiosis in reptiles. Sem Avian Exot Pet Med 2003;12:49–56.

[32] Ladds PW, Mangunwirjo H, Sebayand D. Diseases of young farmed crocodiles in Irian Jaya. Vet Rec 1995;136:121–4.

[33] Taylor MA, Geach MR, Cooley WA. Clinical and pathological observations on natural infections of cryptosporidiosis and flagellate protozoa in leopard geckos (*Eublepharis macularus*). Vet Rec 1999;145:695–9.

[34] Graczyk TK, Blazs GH, Work T, et al. *Cryptosporidium* sp. infection in green turtles, *Chelonia mydas*, as a potential source of marine waterborne cysts in the Hawaiian Islands. Appl Environ Microbiol 1997;63:2925–7.

[35] Cranfield MR, Graczyk TK, Bostwick EF. A comparative assessment of therapeutic efficacy of hyperimmune bovine colostrums treatment against *Cryptosporidium* infection in leopard geckos, *Eublepharis macularus*, and savannah monitors, *Varanus exanthematicus*. Proc ARAV, Columbus, OH; 1999. p. 119–21.

[36] Schell SC. Trematodes of North America north of Mexico. Moscow (ID): University of Idaho Press; 1965. p. 263.

[37] Schmidt GD. CRC handbook of tapeworm identification. Boca Raton (FL): CRC Press; 1984. p. 675.

[38] Khalil LF, Jones A. Keys to the cestode parasites of vertebrates. Wallingford (England): CAB International; 1994. p. 751.

[39] Lane TJ, Mader DR. Parasitology. In: Mader DR, editor. Reptile medicine and surgery. Philadelphia (PA): WB Saunders; 1996. p. 125–40.

[40] Bodri MS. Common parasitic diseases of reptiles and amphibians. In: Proceedings of the Annual Conference of the Association of Reptilian and Amphibian Veterinarians. Pittsburgh (PA): Association of Reptilian and Amphibian Veterinarians; 1994. p. 11–7.

[41] Marcus LC. Veterinary biology and medicine of captive amphibians and reptiles. Philadelphia (PA): Lea & Febiger; 1981.

VETERINARY
CLINICS
Exotic Animal Practice

ELSEVIER
SAUNDERS

Vet Clin Exot Anim 8 (2005) 299–306

Diagnosis and Management of *Macrorhabdus ornithogaster* (Formerly Megabacteria)

David Phalen, DVM, PhD, DABVP-Avian[a,b,*]

[a]*Schubot Exotic Bird Health Center, Veterinary Pathobiology, College of Veterinary Medicine, Texas A&M University, College Station, TX 77843-4467*
[b]*Department of Large Animal Clinical Sciences, College of Veterinary Medicine, Texas A&M University, College Station, TX 77843-4475, USA*

Definition and historical perspective

Key to understanding *Macrorhabdus ornithogaster* is knowing what it is. When it was first described, it was recognized correctly as being a yeast. It stained with silver stains and the periodic acid-Schiff stain (PAS), both of which stain fungi [1,2]. Because of its unusual long, slender shape, however, subsequent investigators could not demonstrate a nucleus or other typical eukaryotic organelles and concluded that it was a bacterium [3]. In 1990, Scanlan and Graham [4] published a paper that indicated that they had isolated the so-called "megabacterium" and that it was a facultative anaerobic and capnophilic bacterium that was sensitive to many antibiotics. The bacterium that they isolated, however, was smaller and more variable in size than the organisms in situ. Additionally, they did not characterize the organism by electron microscopy, they failed to show whether their isolate stained with PAS or silver stains, and they did not attempt to reproduce the disease by infecting budgerigars. Other investigators subsequently isolated similar bacteria from the proventriculus of the budgerigar and ostriches and assumed that these were the so-called "megabacteria" [5–7]. Additional work with these bacterial isolates led to the erroneous conclusion that the so-called "megabacteria" can infect mammals [8–11].

Realization that the so-called "megabacteria" were, in fact, a fungus came in several steps. Initially, not all investigators were able to grow a bacterium from the proventriculus of infected birds, even when large

---

* Department of Large Animal Clinical Sciences, College of Veterinary Medicine, Texas A&M University, College Station, TX 77843-4475, USA.
  E-mail address: dphalen@cvm.tamu.edu

doi:10.1016/j.cvex.2004.12.002
vetexotic.theclinics.com

numbers of organisms were present. Gerlach [12] was able to isolate an organism with the appropriate morphology using a fungal medium; however, the isolate only could be passaged for a few times before it would no longer grow. Subsequently, it was shown to grow slowly in cell culture media that was supplemented with dextrose, fetal calf serum, and antibacterial antibiotics [13]. Filippich and Perry [14] used infected birds to show that the so-called "megabacteria" were not susceptible to antibiotics and were only susceptible to amphotericin B. German and American investigators showed that the organism stained with blancophor BA and calcofluor white M2R—stains that are specific for keratin and cellulose, which are found only in eukaryotes [15,16]. Proof that this organism was a yeast came when German investigators were able to demonstrate that it had a nucleus on electron microscopy and that it contained eukaryotic ribosomal DNA [13]. Tomaszewski et al [16] purified the organism and sequenced the DNA coding for the ribosomal RNA. This information proved that the so-called "megabacterium" was not a bacterium, but a previously undescribed yeast which they named *Macrorhabdus ornithogaster*. *Macrorhabdus ornithogaster* is Greek for a "long rod from a bird's stomach." It is a member of the phylum Ascomycetes and is the only species in its unique genus.

Affected species and clinical manifestations of disease

M ornithogaster was first recognized in the early 1980s [1,3,17]. Where it originated and whether it was present in aviculture and wild birds before this is not known. It has a worldwide distribution, has been found in wild and companion species of birds, and is believed to be increasingly prevalent [12,18]. The potential host range of *M ornithogaster* seems to be extensive and ranges from parrots and finches to ducks and ibis [1,2,19–22]. The significance of this organism in many of these species should be interpreted conservatively, because in many cases, little information on how these organisms were identified was provided. Just because this organism has been reported in a species, it does not mean that it is common in that species or that it has been associated with disease in that species. The prevalence of infection in budgerigar, parrotlet, canary, and finch aviaries often is high [1,6,15,17,23].

It is increasingly clear that *M ornithogaster*, under certain poorly-defined circumstances, is a pathogen [18]. It is equally clear that infection with *M ornithogaster*, under most circumstances, does not result in disease; detection of the organism in a sick or dead bird does not prove that it was the cause of the bird's illness. Factors that may predispose to *M ornithogaster*–associated disease include a genetic predisposition of the host; management issues, such as crowding and hygiene; and possibly, variation in strains of *M ornithogaster* [14,18,23].

An acute and chronic form of *M ornithogaster*–associated disease has been described. In the acute presentation, apparently healthy birds suddenly go off feed, regurgitate ingesta that may be blood stained, and die within 1 to 2 days. This form of disease may be the typical presentation in parrotlets and is an uncommon presentation in budgerigars [19,24]. In the more common chronic form, affected birds seem to be hungry and spend a lot of time at the food dish. Instead of eating, however, these birds are grinding their food but not ingesting it. Regurgitation is common and fresh or dried saliva is found often on the tops of affected birds' heads. Undigested seeds may be present in the droppings. Diarrhea with or without melena also may be present. These birds go through a prolonged period of weight loss (going light) where they appear unthrifty and eventually die [17,19]. Typically, in large budgerigar aviaries that are experiencing this problem, there always will be a few birds that show these signs. Birds that have clinical signs of infection are reported to have decreased packed cell volumes and low sodium, chloride, phosphate, glucose, cholesterol, and aspartate aminotransferase values [25]. When there was gastric ulceration, markedly decreased total protein concentrations were observed. Contrast radiography revealed, in some birds, a dilated proventriculus and an increased transit time. Mature birds were affected most commonly with a mean age of 2.7 years in one aviary [19,20]. Other diseases in budgerigars also can cause similar signs; these include candidiasis of the crop or ventriculus, a bacterial ventriculitis, trichomoniasis, enteritis, heavy metal poisoning, and neoplasia of the stomach. Most infections in budgerigars, and probably in other species of birds, never cause disease. The author has monitored birds in his aviary and found significant numbers of *M ornithogaster* in up to 70% of the budgerigars, yet there was no associated disease.

A chronic form of the disease also seems to occur in canaries, finches, and ostriches. The disease in canaries and finches probably is similar to the chronic form that is seen in budgerigars [1,3,20]. Because these birds tend to hide their illness, however, most bird owners first recognize that there is a problem when an emaciated bird is found dead [3,24]. Reported cases in ostriches occurred in 10-day to 12-week-old chicks. Birds appeared normal but ceased growing and lost weight. Eventually, they became weak and died. Birds had soiled vents and were anemic. Diarrhea was observed in some birds, whereas others had dry, pelleted stools. Mortality rates varied from 40% to 80% in affected flocks [5].

There are three reports of naturally-occurring *M ornithogaster* infections in gallinaceous birds. All three of these reports described infections in chickens (*Gallus gallus domesticus*) and one reported infection in the Japanese quail (*Couturnix japonica*) [26–28]. In the first report, birds were stunted and prone to eat litter and pick each other. The latter two studies described flocks that were affected by multiple pathogens; it was not clear to what extent *M ornithogaster* contributed to the observed morbidity and mortality [27,28]. Chickens that were infected experimentally with *M ornithogaster* did not develop clinical signs of disease; however, the feed conversion rate in infected birds was reduced compared with noninfected controls. This suggested that *M ornithogaster* may have an important economic significance if introduced into poultry flocks [29].

Antemortem and postmortem detection of *Macrorhabdus ornithogaster*

M ornithogaster is a long, straight, narrow rod with rounded ends. It is 2 μm to 4 μm wide and 20 μm to 80 μm long (Figs. 1 and 2). Occasionally, it has a single Y-shaped branch at one end. The longer organisms are actually chains of two to four cells, but the septations between cells are not observed readily. They are gram-positive, but many organisms will not pick up the stain; when they do, only the cytoplasm stains, the thick cell wall does not. Similarly, *M ornithogaster* stains poorly and variably with quick stains that are used for cytology [16]. It is the author's impression that the organism is washed off slides easily during the staining process.

Antemortem diagnosis is done most commonly by microscopic examination of the droppings. The easiest way to do this is to make a wet mount of a fresh dropping and examine it under 40× magnification with the stage condenser almost completely closed. If birds are shedding significant numbers of *M ornithogaster*, they will be readily visible and infection can be confirmed. Many, probably most, sick birds that have macrorhabdosis will shed large numbers of organisms in their droppings. The number of organisms that is shed in the droppings from an asymptomatically infected bird can vary from many to none. Examining five droppings from each bird will increase the chance of finding *M ornithogaster* and also increases the chance of finding fecal debris that can look remarkably like *M ornithogaster*. If there is some uncertainty as to whether a dropping contains *M ornithogaster*, a fecal smear can be stained with calcofluor M2R [18,24]. Dr. Karen Snowden (ksnowden@cvm.tamu.edu) at Texas A&M offers this stain. Staining slides with a Gram stain or a quick stain also may identify the

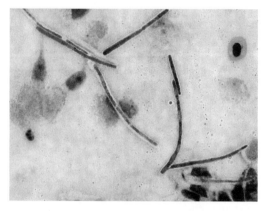

Fig. 1. *Macrorhabdus ornithogaster* stained with the Gram's stain (original magnification ×100). Note the characteristic rod-shape, rounded ends, and thick cell walls. Only the cytoplasm stains and it stains with variable intensity.

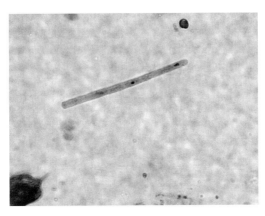

Fig. 2. *Macrorhabdus ornithogaster* stained with the Geimsa stain (original magnification ×100). The dense blue structures within the cytoplasm are the nuclei.

organism, if the wet mount yields questionable results. Stained fecal debris also can resemble *M ornithogaster*. Because not all infected birds shed *M ornithogaster* in their droppings, fecal examination cannot be used to rule out infection.

Postmortem diagnosis of *M ornithogaster* infection is made readily. The proventriculus and ventriculus should be cut in half longitudinally. One half can be formalin fixed. The second half is scraped with a scalpel blade at the junction between the proventriculus and ventriculus (the isthmus). If the organisms are present they will be visible in a wet mount of the scrapings. Grossly, birds that have *M ornithogaster*–associated disease have been described as having a distended proventriculus that is lined by a thick layer of mucus. There may be gross changes in the koilin; in severe cases, the koilin or proventricular mucosa may be ulcerated. Histologically, the organisms are palely eosinophilic and are present at the tips of the glands of the isthmus lined up in parallel, like logs in a log jam. They can be seen better in Gram-, PAS-, or silver-stained sections. In more severe cases, the number of organisms increases and they move into the spaces between the glands and will be seen on the surface of the koilin of the gizzard, and, at times, invade it. Atrophy of the glands of the isthmus and ulceration of the isthmus and koilin develop in the most severe cases. Before ulceration, there may be little or no inflammation. When inflammation does occur, it typically is a lymphoplasmacytic infiltration of the lamina propria of the glands of the isthmus. A moderate thickening of the lamina propria of the isthmus glands was noted in chickens that were infected experimentally with *M ornithogaster*. Dilation of the proventricular glands and disruption of the normal structure of the koilin are other lesions that may be seen [1–3,6,15,17,19,23].

Organisms that resemble *M ornithogaster* have been described in the intestines, and in the liver, in rare cases [12]. Details of how these organisms were characterized were not provided. In the future, *M ornithogaster*–like organisms that are seen outside of the stomach need to be characterized by special staining to prove that they are what they appear to be.

Often, it is difficult to know if the presence of the *M ornithogaster* is sufficient evidence to conclude that the bird died from this infection. This is especially the case in budgerigars in which infections are common, but disease is rare. Ultimately, a decision regarding the importance of an infection will need to be made based on a combination of history, severity of the infection and associated lesions, and the presence or absence of other diseases in the bird.

Treating *Macrorhabdus ornithogaster*

Initial reports that suggested that the so-called "megabacteria" were sensitive to antibiotics are incorrect, because the isolates that were being tested were bacteria and were not the organism that we now know to be *M ornithogaster* [4]. Originally, nystatin was believed to be an effective treatment for *M ornithogaster*, but was not proved to be in subsequent investigations [14]. Fluconazole showed some promise in experimentally-infected chickens, but was found to be toxic in budgerigars at a daily dosage of 10 mg/kg; even at this concentration it was not effective at killing the organism. Iodine preparations, luphenuron, ketoconazole, terbinafine, and itraconazole also were not effective against *M ornithogaster* in other trials [14,24]. Amphotericin B is the only antimicrobial that is effective against *M ornithogaster* [24]. Treatment was effective when it was given at a dosage of 100 mg/kg by gavage twice a day for 30 days. A water-soluble preparation (Megabac-S, Vetafarm, Wagga Wagga, Australia), when given for 14 days, was not effective [24]. A strain of *M ornithogaster* that is resistant to amphotericin B was identified in Australia [14]. It is not known how widespread resistance to amphotericin B may be. It is possible that the water-soluble form of amphotericin may work on other strains or may be more effective if given for longer periods of time.

M ornithogaster shedding ceased when a *Lactobacillus* sp was administered by gavage in treated budgerigars [21]. The birds were not necropsied, so it is not known if they were cured or just stopped shedding the organism temporarily. It was suggested that macrorhabdosis results in an increased pH of the proventriculus, but this has not been verified by other investigators. It was suggested that decreasing the pH of the stomach may be a useful treatment, but this hypothesis remains unproven.

Evidence suggests that there are mixed benefits to treating an entire flock of birds for *M ornithogaster*. It requires that amphotericin B be given by gavage to every bird twice a day for 30 days. Additionally, it requires that the environment be cleaned extensively and disinfected; we do not know which disinfectants are effective against *M ornithogaster*. With these constraints, flock treatment is not likely to result in a flock cure. Filippich and Perry [14], however, suggested that treatment with the water-soluble amphotericin resulted in a significant reduction in the birds that were shedding the organism. Culling positive birds without treatment did not result in a reduction of shedding; however, it was suggested that culling positive birds after treatment may be of some benefit because these birds may be infected with amphotericin-resistant strains.

An alternate approach to eliminating the infection from a flock is the use of incubator hatching and hand-raising the young. Experimentally, it was shown that if budgerigar eggs are pulled from the parents and cleaned and the chicks are not allowed to have contact with the egg or infected birds after hatching, infection does not occur [30]. Hand-feeding nestling day-old parrotlets and budgerigars and keeping them isolated from other birds is not an easy task; however, a breeder may be willing to do this if this organism is a problem in a flock of valuable breeding birds.

References

[1] Dorrestein GM, Zwart P, Buitellaar MN. Problems arising from disease during the periods of breeding and rearing canaries and other aviary birds. Tijdschr Diergeneeskd 1980;105: 535–43.

[2] Hargreaves RC. A fungus commonly found in the proventriculus of small pet birds. In: 30th Western Poultry Disease Conference and 15th Poultry Health Symposium. Davis (CA): University of California at Davis; 1981. p. 75–6.

[3] van Herck H, Duijser T, Zwart P, et al. A bacterial proventriculitis of canaries. Avian Pathol 1984;13:561–72.

[4] Scanlan CM, Graham DL. Characterization of a gram-positive bacterium from the proventriculus of budgerigars (*Melopsittacus undulatus*). Avian Dis 1990;34:779–86.

[5] Huchzermeyer FW, Henton MM, Keffen RH. High mortality associated with megabacteriosis of proventriculus and gizzard in ostrich chicks. Vet Rec 1993;133:143–4.

[6] Simpson VR. Megabacteriosis in exhibition budgerigars. Vet Rec 1992;131:203–4.

[7] Rossi G. Histological and immunohistochemical findings in proventricular mucosa of chickens experimentally infected with "megabacterium." In: Proceeding of the 18th Meeting of the European Society of Veterinary Pathology. Grugliasco, Italy; 2000. p. 156.

[8] Rossi G. Possibility of infecting mammals with megabacteria isolated from birds. Vet Rec 2000;147:371.

[9] Ross G. Possibility of infecting mammals with megabacteria from birds. Vet Rec 2000;146: 444.

[10] Huchzermyer F, Henton NM. Megabacteria in mammals. Vet Rec 2000;146:768.

[11] Cooke SW. Role of megabacteria in mammals. Vet Rec 2000;147:371–2.

[12] Gerlach H. Megabacteriosis. Sem Avian Exotic Pet Med 2001;10:12–9.

[13] Ravelhofer-Rotheneder K, Engelhardt H, Wolf O, et al. Taxonomic classification of "megabacteria" isolates originating from budgerigars (*Melopsittacus undulatus*). Tierarztl Prax 2000;28:415–20.

[14] Filippich LJ, Perry RA. Drug trials against Megabacteria in budgerigars (*Melopsittacus undulatus*). Aust Vet Practit 1993;23:184–9.

[15] Ravelhofer K, Rotheneder R, Gareis M, et al. Megabacteriosis in different bird species [German]. DVG Tag Vogelkr 1998;9:95–104.

[16] Tomaszewski EK, Logan KE, Kurtzman CP, Snowden KF, Phalen DN. Phylogenetic analysis indicates the "megabacterium" of birds is a novel anamorphic ascomycetous yeast, *Macrorhabdus ornithogaster*, gen. nov., sp. nov. Int J Sys Evol Micro 2003;3:1201–5.

[17] Baker JR. Clinical and pathological aspects of "going light" in exhibition budgerigars (*Melopsittacus undulatus*). Vet Rec 1985;116:406–8.

[18] Antinoff N, Filippich LJ, Speer B, et al. Diagnosis and treatment options for megabacteria (*Macrorhabdus ornithogaster*). J Avian Med Surg 2004;18:189–95.

[19] Filippich LJ, O'Boyle DA, Webb R, et al. Megabacteria in birds in Australia. Aust Vet Prac 1993;23:72–6.

[20] Filippich LJ, Parker MG. Megabacteriosis and proventricular/ventricular disease in psittacines and passerines. In: Proceedings of the Annual Conference of the Association of Avian Veterinarians. Reno (NV): Association of Avian Veterinarians; 1994. p. 287–93.

[21] Lublin A. A five-year survey of megabacteriosis in birds of Israel and a biological control. In: Proceedings of the Annual Conference of the Association of Avian Veterinarians. St Paul (MN): Association of Avian Veterinarians; 1998. p. 241–5.

[22] Pennycott TW, Ross HM, McLaren IM, et al. Causes of death of wild birds of the family Fringillidae in Britain. Vet Rec 1998;143:155–8.

[23] Fillippich LJ, Herdrikz JK. Prevalence of megabacteria in budgerigar colonies. Aust Vet J 1998;76:92–5.

[24] Phalen DN, Tomaszewski E, Davis A. Investigation into the detection, treatment, and pathogenicty of avian gastric yeast. In: Proceedings of the 23rd Annual Conference of the Association of Avian Veterinarians. Monterey (CA): Association of Avian Veterinarians; 2002. p. 49–51.

[25] Henderson GM, Gulland MD, Hawkey CM. Haematological findings in budgerigars with megabacterium and trichomonas infections associated with 'going light.' Vet Rec 1988;123: 492–4.

[26] Mutlu OF, Seckin S, Ravelhofer SK, et al. Proventriculitis in fowl caused by megabacteria. Tierarztl Prax 1997;25:460–2.

[27] Schulze C, Heidrich R. Megabacteria-associated proventriculitis in poultry in the state of Brandenburg, Germany. Dtsch Tierärztl Wochenschr 2001;108:264–6.

[28] Pennycott TW, Duncan G, Venugopal K. Marek's disease, candidiasis and megabacteriosis in a flock of chickens (*Gallus gallus domesticus*) and Japanese quail (*Coturnix japonica*). Vet Rec 2003;153:293–7.

[29] Phalen DN, Moore R. Experimental infection of white-leghorn cockerels with *Macrorhabdus ornithogaster* (Megabacterium). Avian Dis 2003;47:254–60.

[30] Moore RP, Snowden KF, Phalen DN. A method of preventing transmission of so-called megabacteria in budgerigars (*Melopsittacus undulatus*). J Avian Med Surg 2001;15:283–7.

ELSEVIER
SAUNDERS

VETERINARY
CLINICS
Exotic Animal Practice

Vet Clin Exot Anim 8 (2005) 307–327

Raptor Gastroenterology

Eric Klaphake, DVM[a],*, Jo Clancy[b]

[a]*The University of Tennessee, Department of Small Animal Clinical Sciences,
College of Veterinary Medicine, C247 Veterinary Teaching Hospital,
Knoxville, TN 37996-4544, USA*
[b]*The University of Tennessee, Office of the Dean, Class 2007, College of Veterinary Medicine
2407 River Drive, Knoxville, TN 37996, USA*

The term "raptor" refers to the carnivorous members of the Orders Falconiformes and Strigiformes, represented by hawks, falcons, caracaras, eagles, ospreys, kites, condors, vultures, secretary birds; and owls, respectively. Although the majority of birds represented in veterinary medicine are of the orders Psittaformes, Galliformes, Passeriformes, and Columbiformes, raptors are a group of birds with some important gastrointestinal (GI) differences. These differences in anatomy, physiology, nutrition, and disease etiologies can greatly effect the direction and the success of medical and surgical intervention of raptor GI diseases. Raptor patients can be a free-living individual, a nonreleasable education animal, a falconry bird, or a display or breeding animal from a zoologic or private institution. Correct diagnosis is as important as successful treatment when considering zoonotic potential and contagious diseases. Because of potential harm from talons, beaks, and even the wings of raptors; hospitalization and long-term management needs to take these risks into account. No raptor species is truly domesticated, so the toll that diagnostics and therapeutics may take on these patients is equally important to consider.

To classify a disease into a single anatomic system such as the GI system is often inaccurate. Likewise, although many diseases enter the body orally, they are systemically absorbed and do not directly affect the GI system. The GI system plays a primary role in a raptor's nutritional status, so conditions such as starvation secondary to a humeral fracture may indirectly involve the GI system. The effects of long-term food deprivation in the cold (5°C) on barn owls (*Tyto alba*) found that body mass and nitrogen loss were kept constant for 7.2 ± 1.6 days [1]. A metabolic shift leading to increased

* Corresponding author.
 E-mail address: eklaphak@utk.edu (E. Klaphake).

nitrogen loss and body mass at 7.9 + 1.7 days found owls still able to fly and to feed themselves. However, the authors felt the a rise in nitrogen loss would precede death from starvation by less than 2.5 days.

The normal diet of free-living raptors varies considerably from species to species, although the vast majority involves other animals [2–4]. Raptors may vary from their reported normal diet to opportunistically presenting items or when current conditions do not allow access to normal prey [5–7]. In captivity, dietary options can be limited. Several studies have evaluated the nutritional content of hamsters, 1-day-old chicks, quail, chickens, rats, and guinea pigs [8,9]. Most items provided adequate amounts of protein, lipid, vitamin A, calcium, magnesium, and zinc; however, deficiencies in vitamin E, copper, iron, and manganese were noted [9].

Retrospective reviews of morbidity and mortality in specific species or in raptors in general puts the involvement of GI disease into perspective. Of 340 raptors admitted and diagnosed at the University of Florida Veterinary Medical Teaching Hospital from 1988 to 1994, 6% presented due to toxicosis, 4% for poor nutrition, and 3% for infectious disease [10]. At an Alabama raptor rehabilitation center, emaciation was the only possible GI disease reason for presentation of a raptor of the five most common causes [11]. Of 163 red-tailed hawks (*Buteo jamaicensis*) presented to the National Wildlife Center from 1975 to 1992, 20% died of emaciation of an unknown etiology, 15% of pesticide exposure, and 13% of infectious etiologies including pox, pasteurellosis, and tuberculosis [12]. Of 132 great horned owls (*Bubo virginianus*) presented to the National Wildlife Center from 1975 to 1993, 20% died of emaciation of an unknown etiology, 8% of pesticide exposure, and 5% of infectious etiologies [13]. In 81 barn owls and five Hawaiian owls (*Asio flammeus sandwichensis*) in Hawaii from 1992 to 1994, 22% died of emaciation of an unknown etiology, 0% of pesticide exposure, and 28% of infectious etiologies including trichomoniasis and pasteurellosis [14]. In 546 golden eagles (*Aquila chrysaetos*) and bald eagles (*Haliaeetus leucocephalus*) in western Canada from 1986 to 1998, 6% died of emaciation of an unknown etiology, 18% of pesticide exposure, and 6% of infectious etiologies including pasteurellosis [15].

Anatomy and physiology of the raptor gastrointestinal system

The GI tract is variable among avian species, including between Falconiformes and Strigiformes. The GI tract is adapted to facilitate flight by minimizing weight and length when compared with mammals. The GI tract of raptors, as in other birds, is centrally located within the body cavity to assist in maintaining balance and aerodynamic ability. There are a greater number of organs within the GI tract of birds, compared with mammals; therefore, there is greater interorgan communication [16]. Species requiring rapid acceleration and maneuverability to capture prey in flight such as the accipiter (*Accipiter* sp.), peregrine falcons (*Falco perigrinus*), and barn owls have the lightest digestive tracts (small intestine, proventriculus, ventriculus, and liver) relative to body size, while raptors not relying on rapid flight acceleration such as the buteos (*Buteo* sp.) and tawny owls (*Strix aluco*) have heavier digestive tracts relative to body size [17]. The GI tract of most avian species is comprised of the beak, oropharynx (mouth, tongue, and pharynx), esophagus, ingluvies (crop), proventriculus, ventriculus (gizzard), intestine, ceca, rectum, cloaca, and vent [18]. Accessory glands to the GI tract include salivary glands, pancreas, liver, and gall bladder. Histologically, the intestinal tract is lined with a continuous mucous membrane from the oropharynx to vent [18]. The epithelial layer consists of the lamina propria, lamina muscularis, and sometimes a submucosa layer, which provide protection from abrasion and invading microorganisms [18]. The primary function of the digestive tract is the absorption of nutrients and the exclusion of nonnutritional elements [18].

The upper gastrointestinal system

The upper and lower mandible of the avian species is covered with a kertatinized sheath, referred to as the rhamphotheca and the gnathotheca, respectively. The shape and size of the beak are adapted for the type of food consumed, and allows for differences in feeding styles. Falcons (*Falco* sp.) have sharp edges on their beak, the tomial tooth, and serrated edges for cutting [19]. The beak is also the entry point of the respiratory system [16], containing the nares on the rhamphotheca. Eurasian kestrels' (*Falco tinnunculus*) method of capturing their prey suggests their bill is not used to kill prey, but to damage the central nervous system to minimize escape attempts [20].

The primary function of the oral cavity is for grasping and the mechanical processing of food, and also for the lubrication and propelling of food into the esophagus [21]. Backward pointing rows of papillae run transversely across the roof and floor of the oral cavity to help direct food during swallowing [22]. The oral cavity and the pharynx are often referred to commonly as the oropharynx [18]. Birds, unlike mammals, lack a soft palate. Most birds do not have overlapping musculature in the tongue [21]. Extrinsic muscles attached to the hyoid apparatus mobilize the tongue [18]. Falconiformes and Strigiformes have a rasp-like surface on the rostral portion of their tongue composed of keratinized stratified squamous epithelium, allowing for greater food manipulation and swallowing ability; however, the tongue has a decreased ability to protrude from the beak and mouth [18]. Mucus-producing salivary glands are located in the walls of the oropharynx but are less developed in Falconiformes and Strigiformes. An evaluation of the usefulness of feeding repellents based on chemical additives affecting taste found some food rejection occurring by American kestrels (*Falco sparverius*), although not to the point of starvation. A second study determined that visual cues were more successful in encouraging food-item rejection [23]. A survey of aerobic bacterial flora from the choana of free-living and captive red-tailed hawks (*Buteo jamaicensis*) and Cooper's hawks (*Accipiter cooperii*) isolated co-agulase-negative *Staphylococcus/Micrococcus* sp. and *Corynebacterium* sp. most frequently in all red-tailed hawks and in free-living Cooper's hawks, with *Pasteurella* sp. and *Corynebacterium* sp. found commonly in captive Cooper's hawks [24]. However, in a study looking specifically for *Pasteurella multocida* in 398 raptors, only birds with clinical disease had positive choanal or pharyngeal cultures [25].

The pharynx joins the esophagus, and extends along the right side of the neck into the thoracic cavity and terminates in the proventriculus. The esophagus is expandable due to longitudinal folds along its entirety. It is lined with incompletely keratinized stratified squamous epithelial cells with subepithelial mucous glands for lubrication [21]. Falconiformes have greater dilation ability compared with Strigiformes, which have no dilation ability of the esophagus (Fig. 1) [26]. The ingluvies (crop) is located cranial to the thoracic inlet, and is a dilation of the esophagus. The ingluvies functions as a temporary food storage unit and to soften food [27]. The ingluvies and esophagus are important in the nourishment of young fledglings. Adult birds will store food to regurgitate to feed to their young. A defining characteristic of a "true crop" is the presence of a controllable sphincter, which regulates the entrance and exit of food [16]. Strigiformes do not possess an ingluvies, but most Falconiformes have well-developed ingluvies [28]. The bearded vulture (*Gypaetus barbatus*) is the only vulture species to lack an ingluvies, instead relying on the esophagus for food storage [29]. To pass food from ingluvies to stomach a Falconiforme will "put over" by stretching the head up, then pushing it chin down first in a flattening movement, often wriggling the head far to one side [22].

The lower gastrointestinal system

The stomach of birds is divided into the glandular stomach (pro-ventriculus) and the muscular stomach (ventriculus or gizzard) [22]. Carnivores and piscivores have a larger proventriculus and often a smaller, weaker, thin-walled ventriculus. The ventriculus functions to mechanically massage and grind food to reduce its size and increase the surface area, although in raptors, the ventriculus is often thin walled and reduced in size [22]. The proventriculus merges into the ventriculus, giving it a pear shape, and is lined with koilin, a proteinaceous, cuticular lining secreted by a layer of mucous glands that protects the ventriculus from acid secreted in the proventriculus [22]. The posterior portion of the ventriculus tapers into

Fig. 1. GI systems of a Falconiformes raptor (*A*) compared with a Strigiformes raptor (*B*) (Courtesy of Jo Clancy). Note absence of the ingluvies in the Strigiformes, the smaller pancreas in the Falconiformes, and the vestigial nature of the caeca in the Falconiformes.

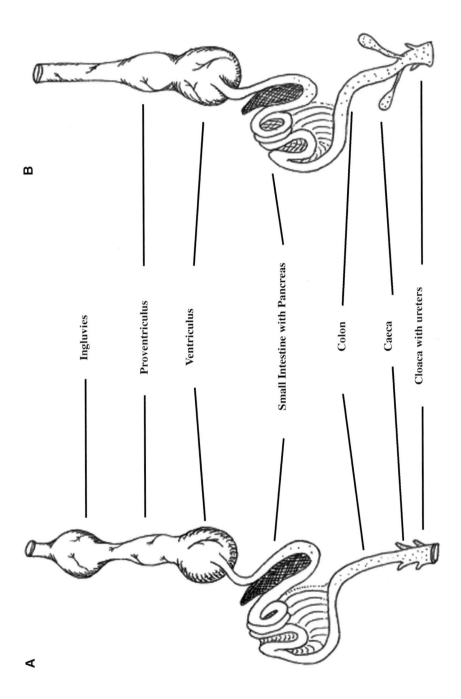

Ingluvies

Proventriculus

Ventriculus

Small Intestine with Pancreas

Colon

Caeca

Cloaca with ureters

A

B

a pyloric region, where the mucosa allows for passage of liquefied digesta into the small intestine, while trapping or filtering undigested food components [21]. The common buzzard (*Buteo buteo*) has a contraction pressure of 8 to 26 mmHg [22]. The pH of the proventriculus during digestion is as low as 1 in Falconiformes and 3 in Strigiformes [19]. Pellets (castings) are formed in the ventriculus. Raptors normally regurgitate pellets, which are composed of the bones, fur, and feathers of their prey [19]. Falconiformes can digest bones of their prey, whereas Strigiformes have decreased digestibility and often pass pellets with complete skeletons. Strigiformes often regurgitate one pellet per prey eaten, whereas Falconiformes often eat more than one meal before casting [26]. Most casts are egested before midmorning at the night perch or postkilling of prey, but before the first feeding of the day [22]. Cast dry matter in red-tailed hawks and great horned owls (*Bubo virginianus*) was 2% to 8% of consumed dry matter [8]. Many biologists have used the remains found in the pellets of owls to determine prey species. However, in barn owls, remains in the pellets were potentially biased toward larger prey as opposed to smaller prey such as insects [30]. With hen harrier (*Circus cyaneus*) pellets from nests overrepresented mammalian prey and underrepresented avian prey. Pellets were useful estimates of prey diversity, but direct observations of feeding habits completed the overall picture [31]. Insect chitin can be found in pellets, with 23.8% and 29.6% of total chitin ingested in American kestrels and eastern screech owls (*Otus asio*), respectively, egested in pellets [32].

The small intestine is responsible for the enzymatic digestion of food and the absorption of end products. The small intestines show less variability between the avian species compared with other organs [18]. The motility responses to fasting of the GI tract of Galliformes (in times of food deprivation, the GI tract maximizes nutritional resources by recycling whatever food still remains within the GI tract via myoelectric spike potential bursts that propagate GI tract movement in an orad diection) seem to be lacking in barred owls (*Strix varia*) [33]. The diet of the bearded vulture consists largely of bone [29]. With a diet of sheep ribs, two bearded vultures had a mean digestive efficiency of 50%, with most digestion occurring within 24 hours. A bone diet may have a higher caloric content compared with an equivalent weight of soft tissue. Because the digestive tract of the bearded vulture lacks an area for mechanical breakdown of food, these birds rely on the high concentration of acid-secreting cells in the proventriculus [29]. As described earlier in American kestrels, some ingested chitin is egested in pellets (23.8%), but 59.2% passes through into the excreta, while the remainder (17.0%) is digested in the lower GI tract [32]. Dietary fat had little effect on anatomy or GI contractions in American kestrels [34]. American kestrels were reported to have enlarged duodenums relative to the size in other raptors. This enlarged duodenal size allows for a unique reflux of duodenal contents associated with every duodenal flux in each gastroduodenal contraction cycle (approximately 3–4/min) for improved mixing of ingesta with digestive secretions, hastening digestion for this small bird with a high metabolic rate [34]. Ceca are paired, blind-ended tubes located at the junction of the ileum and rectum, responsible for bacterial decomposition of crude fiber in herbivorous birds. The ceca of Falconiformes are vestigial (~4 mm long), while in Strigiformes are large and well developed (Fig. 1) [22]. The colon was relatively larger also in American kestrels [34]. The colon plays an important role in the reabsorption of water [21]. Raptor stool should be formed with black fecal center and surrounded by watery white urates. Emerald green feces can be normal due to unused bile, and is seen a few hours before feeding when the GI system is otherwise empty [35].

A survey of aerobic bacterial flora from the cloaca of free-living and captive red-tailed hawks and Cooper's hawks isolated coagulase-negative *Staphylococcus* sp., *Micrococcus* sp. and *Streptococcus* sp. most frequently in all red-tailed hawks, coagulase-negative *Staphylococcus/Micrococcus* sp. and *Escherichia* sp. in free-living Cooper's hawks. *Escherichia* sp., coagulase-positive *Staphylococcus* sp. and *Streptococcus* sp. Were found commonly in captive Cooper's hawks [24]. *Salmonella* sp. was isolated in free-living birds of both species, but not captive birds; and *Pasteurella* sp. was not isolated from the cloaca of any birds [24]. In a study looking specifically culturing for *Pasteurella multocida* in 398 raptors, only birds with clinical disease had positive cloacal cultures [25]. An evaluation of northern harriers (*Circus cyaneus*) and barn owls for *Salmonella* sp. in feces, found 2 or 19 harriers and 0 of 17 barn owls grew *Salmonella enteriditis*, with the harrier serotype being Montevideo [36]. However, a captive breeding center in Italy had several cases of embryonic and neonatal deaths in European eagle owls (*Bubo bubo*), peregrine falcons, common buzzards, and lanner falcons (*Falco biarmicus*), with *Salmonella havana* and *S. virchow* isolated [37]. Several other *Salmonella* sp. were isolated in the same collection over several years in both healthy, nonclinical birds, and was a cause of morbidity and mortality in others. Raptors have been implicated along with other avian species as potential reservoirs of *Campylobacter* spp. in their intestinal tracts [38]. A report of *Cryptococcus neoformans* in the feces of two healthy eagle owls suggests shedding can occur in these species and proper precautions should be taken for immunocompromised individuals around raptors [39].

Accessory organs

The accessory organs to the GI tract include the pancreas, liver, and gallbladder. The pancreas is located within the duodenal loop and extends half the length of the duodenal loop in Strigiformes, and is even smaller in Falconiformes (Fig. 1) [26]. It is tri-lobed, consisting of the dorsal, ventral, and splenic lobes [18]. The pancreas drains by one to three ducts into the ascending duodenum. Pancreatic enzymes are responsible for the assistance of chemical digestion (amylase, proteases, and trypsin). Alkalines are also produced by the pancreas to neutralize stomach acid [22]. The liver is bilobed and overlies the ventriculus. The liver is larger in raptors compared with other avian species [22]. In the common buzzard, the liver and gall bladder weigh about 20 g—2.5% of total body weight [22]. The liver functions in metabolizing and storing sugars, fats, and vitamins; synthesizing proteins, bile salts and acids; and controlling excretion and detoxification of waste products in the blood. The gall bladder is located on the ventral surface of the right lobe of the liver [21]. It is absent in many species, including some peregrine falcons [22]. The gall bladder collects and stores bile from the liver, and empties via two ducts into the duodenum [21]. Secretion from the gall bladder is continuous and important in carnivorous birds, as it is responsible for the emulsion of fats [22].

Diseases syndromes

Upper gastrointestinal diseases

In raptors, the beak has a key role in killing prey, prehension, and tearing of food. Therefore, disease or damage to the beak can lead to GI problems. A normal, healthy beak should wear evenly in the bird; however, in captivity; raptors may require routine beak maintenance, called "coping" by falconers. Recognizing normal conformation of the beak for each species is important during beak coping. A multispeed rotary tool (Dremel, Dremel Corp., Racine, Wisconson) can be used for routine or therapeutic trimming. Clinical signs of beak disease include: abnormal beak conformation, emaciation, regurgitation, anorexia, and reduced fecal production. Etiologies of beak disease include trauma, developmental abnormalities, nutritional, metabolic, infectious disease, and neoplasia [40]. Raptors often experience trauma, and may be hit by cars, fly into windows, and be attacked by prey or other predators. Malformations of the beak may also occur in raptors that fly into aviary wires [41]. With captive raptors, trauma can be more quickly addressed than in free-living raptors. Management of beak damage is similar to that described in psittacine birds [42]. Congenital beak problems are extremely rare in raptors [42]. Neoplastic disease of the beak may occur, but has been rarely reported in raptors. Incorrect feeding practices can lead to overgrowth of the upper beak, as is seen in raptors on a diet of exclusively soft day-old chicks [41]. Such overgrowth can lead to a fracture of the beak with bleeding and discomfort, or may interfere with normal beak closure. Falcons' tomial teeth on the lateral surfaces of the rhamphoteca can overgrow [22]. An ill-fitted falconry hood can cause pressure necrosis on the germinal tissue of the beak [41]. Change to a properly fitted hood and wound management can be corrective. Hypovitaminosis A can cause dry hyperkeratotic lesions similar to those seen with mites [41]. Dietary or parenteral supplementation with vitamin A is corrective, although dosing should not induce hypervitaminosis

A. Metabolic bone diseases can create severe beak abnormalities [41]. Dietary correction and supplementation may prevent further progression of the abnormalities, but rarely corrects them. Epidermoptid mites (*Knemidocoptes* sp.) have been reported to cause beak lesions [41]. Long-term treatment with ivermectin can be used to try to clear the infection.

Clinical signs of oropharyngeal disease include dyspnea, head shaking, flicking of food, unproductive head and neck movements for aborad food movement, regurgitation, anorexia, emaciation, and scant fecal production [35]. Etiologic categories of oropharyngeal disease include trauma, toxin, neoplasia, nutritional, and infectious causes [40].

Trichomoniasis

Trichomoniasis is one of the major infectious diseases affecting raptors, particularly those feeding on avian prey [35]. The causative organism is a pear-shaped protozoa with several anterior flagella and a trailing flagellum. In a group of 110 nestling Cooper's hawks from North Dakota, Wisconsin, and British Columbia only 2.7% had no signs of mortality in the nestlings due to Trichomonas gallinae infection [43]. Another study of Cooper's hawks in Arizona of 223 nestlings found the prevalence of *Trichomonas gallinae* was 85% in urban nestlings but only 9% in nonurban nestlings [44]. However, in a study of Bonelli's eagles (*Hieraaetus fasciatus*) in Spain, 36% of nestlings had *Trichomonas gallinae*, leading to death in 2% of the chicks [45]. An epiornitic in 1997 in American kestrels and Eastern screech owls was reported in Colorado, with 42 and two birds, respectively, involved [46]. During a 5-year period, 5.5% of all falcons (7085 birds) presented to a falcon specialist veterinary hospital in Saudi Arabia were diagnosed with *Trichomonas gallinae* infection [47]. However, during a 6-year period, 31.2% of falcons (5360 birds) presented to a falcon specialist hospital in Bahrain were diagnosed with *Trichomonas gallinae* infection [48]. Caseous lesions of varying size and location are found around and under the tongue, on the palate, occasionally extending into the ingluvies or the respiratory system [19]. Occasionally a systemic form has been noted [41]. One of the first reported diseases in veterinary medicine, "frounce" is widely distributed throughout the world [49]. The flagellated protozoa are transmitted directly through contact or by ingestion of contaminated food (pigeons and doves are often inapparent carriers) or water. Freezing of pigeons for greater than 24 hours seems to kill or render the parasite innocuous [49]. *Trichomonas gallinae* has been described as a facultatively pathogenic mucosal organism, present in healthy birds, but causing disease with an upper GI injury, immunosuppression, or in younger animals; with goshawks, sparrow hawks, and falcons seeming to be more susceptible [41]. Diagnosis is through identification of the motile trophozoite on immediate cytology with sterile saline [41]. Recommended treatment includes nutritional and fluid supportive care, along with flushing of the lesions with sterile saline and either chlorhexidine gluconate or povidone-iodine for up to 2 weeks as needed [49]. Confirmed or suspected involvement of additional GI organs supports the use of metronidazole (100 mg/kg by mouth every 24 hours for 3 days) [47]. An alternative treatment is carnidazole (30 mg/kg by mouth every 12 hours for 3–5 days) with lesions usually disappearing within 24 to 48 hours [19]. Secondary infection with *Pseudomonas aeruginosa* in captive Saker falcons (*Falco cherrug*) was managed with the addition of pipercillin (100 mg/kg intramuscularly every 12 hours for 7 days) and tobramycin (10 mg/kg intramuscularly every 12 hours for 7 days) and a 1% povidone-iodine mouthwash [50].

Candida albicans *infection*

In a retrospective review of 3760 falcons, 0.3% had candidiasis, also known as "thrush" [51]. *Candida albicans* was the most commonly identified yeast involved, an opportunistic organism that is usually endogenous in origin, with infection triggered by immunosuppression, inadequate nutrition, long-term antibiotic use, or stress [51]. The disease tends to afflict the upper GI system. Endoscopic examination of the upper GI tract may show a "Turkish towel" appearance to the growths on the mucosa. Cytologic examination of lesions with Gram's stain can suggest a yeast component, although microbiological culture is important for species identification and sensitivity. Use of commercially available kits used in human medicine has been reported to be successful [51]. Treatment includes supportive care and the application of a miconazole human oral gel applied liberally with cotton-tipped applicators onto the affected mucosa every 12 hours for 5 days [51]. Other suggested treatments include nystatin topically (200,000–300,000 IU/kg twice a day for 5–7 days) and itraconazole (5–10 mg/kg by mouth twice a day for 7–21 days).

Nematodes infection (Capillaria)

Another oropharyngeal disease reported in raptors is capillariasis. These nematodes can have a direct or indirect (earthworms) life cycle, dependent on the species, with a prepatent period of 3 to 4 weeks. *Capillaria* sp. eggs can be detected in feces or cytology of oropharyngeal masses. Capillariasis-caused abscesses frequently develop into crop fistulae in the ingluvies and esophagus [41]. Environmental and dietary modifications (gulls and crows are purported to be more commonly infected), routine fecals, and use of appropriate anthelmintic medications can prevent or treat capillariasis [41,52]. Poxviruses been reported in free-living and captive raptor populations, excepting those of the Order Strigiformes [53–56]. Although primarily a dermatologic disease, and generally mild and self-limiting in raptors, the diphtheritic form may cause oropharyngeal or esophageal lesions [53]. Similarly, lesions around the beak may prevent normal mastication [53].

Other oropharyngeal diseases reported in raptors include a sinew or tendon wrapped around the tongue [19,57], congenital palate/tongue/beak deformities [57], a proliferative stomatitis in a bearded vulture [58] of suspected viral etiology, an ulcerative stomatitis in a bearded vulture [58], trauma and secondary abscessation due to sharp bones or feathers, tongue bone fractures due to trauma [41], and numerous neoplasias [59]. Neoplasias included a salivary gland adenocarcinoma in an unspecified raptor, squamous cell carcinoma of the palate of an unspecified raptor, pharyngeal epidermoid carcinoma in a red-tailed hawk, and ingluvial (3) and oropharyngeal (1) papillomas of unknown etiology in unspecified raptors, but all surgically removed successfully [59]. Unique esophageal and oropharyngeal abscesses in addition to septicemia-related lesions in hawks due to avian cholera (*Pasteurella multocida*) were reported and not seen in birds of the Order Strigiformes of Family Falconidae [24]. Most of the isolates of eight positive raptors were of somatic serotype 1. All were susceptible to penicillin G, sulfisoxazole, teracycle, and trimethorpim-sulfamethoxazole [60].

Other esophageal and ingluvies diseases reported in raptors include trapped food items, inflammatory stricture of the esophagus [19], over-heating of diets for raptor chicks or diseased/weak birds, cold meat being retained in the ingluvies, with both of the latter potentially leading to ingluvial fistulaes [41]. Fistulaes and esophageal/ingluvial foreign bodies should be managed surgically as previously described [61]. Ingluvial stasis or "sour crop" can be due to a primary bacterial infection from contaminated food, candidiasis, trichomoniasis, systemic ileus, or secondary to nutritional depletion (low condition) [19]. Treatment focuses on treating the underlying cause and nutritional and fluid support.

Lower gastrointestinal diseases

The lower GI tract begins with the proventriculus and terminates with the cloaca and vent. Clinical signs of lower GI disease include abnormal color of urates, polyuria, vomiting, diarrhea, melena, hematochezia, undigested food in the feces, scant feces, and anorexia [40]. Etiologies for lower GI diseases include infection (viral, bacterial, fungal, parasitic), metabolic (hepatic, renal, pancreatic), toxic, foreign bodies, neoplasia, trauma, nutritional, food allergies, antibiotics, behavioral, and reproductive [40]. Motion sickness causing vomiting has been reported in peregrine falcons [19]. Diseases of the proventriculus and ventriculus are not commonly reported in raptors. Mortality in a free-living Mauritius kestrel nestling was due to ventricular impaction [57]. A perforating proventricular ulcer was reported as the cause of death in a bearded vulture [58]. GI foreign bodies were also reported as causes of mortality in bearded vultures (a piece of rubber, a branch, and a wirebrush) [58].

Endoparasites are common in wild raptors; however, most do not generally contribute significantly to morbidity or mortality [62–71]. Enteric parasites can become significant if the bird is subjected to excessive stress or disease [68]. Coccidiosis is considered to be a possible etiology with clinical signs of anorexia or vomiting [19]. Malabsorption secondary to ventricular nematodiasis was believed to be the cause of death in a Japanese mountain hawk eagle (*Spizaetus nipalensis*) with crypt, lamina propria, muscular, and serosal invasion [72]. For treating many endoparasites, as well as ectoparasites, ivermectin may be used. An evaluation of its use in hybrid falcons (*Falco* sp) suggested that a dosage of 2 to 3 mg/kg was safe and effective and successful in treating certain parasitic infections; however, clinical signs suggesting toxicity were seen at 6 to 11 mg/kg dosages [73].

Paramyxovirus

Certain strains of Newcastle disease virus (NDV-avian paramyxovirus serotype I) can cause severe GI disease in certain raptor species [74] Clinical signs reported in raptors include vomiting, anorexia, and central nervous system signs [75]. Species reported to be affected included peregrine, saker, barbary (*Falco cherrug*), and hybird falcons; gyrfalcons (*F rusticolus*), northern goshawk (*Accipiter gentilis*), Eurasian kestrels, common barn owl, tawny owl, black kite (*Milvus migrans*), and common buzzard [75]. Virus was isolated from intestinal, visceral, cloacal, hepatic swabs. Conclusions were that raptors reared and housed in contact with wild birds, pigeons, and poultry (alive or as food) were a consistent finding in outbreaks [75]. A study in free-living raptors in Germany found 2% of diurnal raptors (346 birds) were seropositive to NDV, while all of the owls (55 birds) were negative [76]. A later study by the same authors evaluated organ samples from 331 raptors, with 5.4% testing positive by polymerase chain reaction for NDV nucleic acids, including 15 barn owls, a tawny owl, a common buzzard, and a European kestrel [77]. An evaluation of 20 free-living and 12 captive Andean condors (*Vultur gryphus*) were all seronegative for NDV [78]. A bearded vulture was found dead with no previous clinical signs, but had hemorrhagic intestines and hepatomegaly [79]. Viral isolation from liver and lungs confirmed the presence of NDV.

Toxin exposure

Toxins can have effects throughout the body, but must initially pass through the GI tract. Fenbendazole toxicity was reported in ten African white-backed vultures (*Gyps africanus*), and three lappet-faced vultures (*Torgos tracheliotus*) at a dose of 47 to 60 mg/kg in the feed for 3 days, with six white-backed and one lappet-faced vultures dying [80]. In this author's experience, oral enrofloxacin has been noted to cause regurgitation or anorexia in some cases, typically several days into its administration. Other veterinarians have noted a similar phenomenon occasionally exhibited in their patients, although this has not been documented in a scientific study (E. Klaphake, personal communication, 2004). Enrofloxacin administered at 15 mg/kg by mouth once in red-tailed hawks and great horned owls maintained theorized therapeutic plasma levels until at least 18 hours postadministration, with a 2- to 8-hour lag to for absorption from the GI tract [81].

Recently, numerous deaths of the Oriental white-backed vulture (*Gyps bengalensis*), the long-billed vulture (*Gyps indicus*), and the slender-billed vulture (*Gyps tenuirostris*), in the Indian subcontinent are believed to be secondary to exposure to the veterinary nonsteroidal anti-inflammatory drug diclofenac in livestock carcasses [82]. Primary toxicity effect causes renal failure in these raptors.

Lead toxicosis is a commonly reported and well-known GI disease in raptors [15,83–90]. In bald and golden eagles in Western Canada from 1986 to 1998, 6.4% of all cases of morbidity or mortality in these species were reported to be due to lead toxicosis [15]. Exposure is usually through ingestion of hunter-injured or killed prey species with residual lead bullets or pellets [85–87]. Another source of concern is the feeding of raptors on urban prey species such as house sparrows (*Passer domesticus*) and pigeons (*Columbia livia*) that may be being exposed to the same environmental sources of lead of concern to humans [91,92]. Turkey vultures have bee noted to be more resistant to lead toxicity [93], although a peripheral neuropathy due to lead toxicosis was reported in a turkey vulture [94]. Clinical signs of lead toxicosis in raptors include ataxia, paresis/paralysis, seizures, lethargy, anorexia, shredding of food, vomiting, weight loss, and lime green feces [89]. Radiographic evidence of metal opacities in the GI tract or high blood lead concentrations supports the diagnosis of lead toxicity. Blood lead concentrations can be submitted to an outside laboratory or run by a veterinarian using an electro-chemical method in-house (LeadCare Blood Lead Testing System, ESA Inc., Chelmsford, Massachusetts) with toxicosis indicated at levels greater than 20 µg/dL (0.20 ppm) [89]. Treatment of lead toxicity includes supportive care, treatment of symptoms, and removal of the lead source. Lead can be removed manually via surgical extraction, gastric lavage, or endoscopy [89]. Lead may be "flushed" through the GI tract with the use of force feeding to physically move the particles; however, with the weight of some particles, they may sink to the bottom of the ventriculus and allow force-fed materials to pass over them. Likewise, because of lead's effect on the nervous system, ileus may prevent flushing from being effective and may instead be detrimental. Lead can also be removed chemically, through the use of the heavy metal chelator calcium disodium ethylenediaminetetracetate (Ca EDTA) at 50 mg/kg intramuscularly every 12 hours for 2–23 days [89]. With Ca EDTA chelation, the mean reduction of blood lead concentrations was 84% [89]. No deleterious effects from use of Ca EDTA were seen in any of the falcons in which it was used [89].

Other ingested or suspected toxins in raptors include environmental contaminants and pesticides [58,95–112], tetrodotoxicosis from ingestion of a California newt (*Taricha torosa*) in a great horned owl [113], and ethylene glycol toxicosis in a California condor (*Gymnogyps californianus*) [114].

Droppings

Stool should be well formed with a dark fecal center and surrounded by watery white urates. Emerald green feces can be normal due to unused bile, and is seen a few hours before feeding when the GI system is otherwise empty [19]. Lime green stool suggest alterations in motility and absorptive processes caused by aspergillosis, lead toxicity, coccidian, anaerobic, or idiopathic GI infection. Jade green stools due to increased biliverdin production from hemolysis may suggest a plasmodial infection of the erythrocytes. Mucus in the stool from severe intestinal insult may be due to a coccidial infection. Granular, yellowish-tinged feces can be due to cloacal uroliths, and a primary cause for those needs to be evaluated. True diarrhea suggests inflammation or infection, often due to coccidiosis or salmonellosis [19]. A rotavirus has been suspected in a group of young merlins (*Falco columbarius*) showing signs of stunted growth and lethargy [54]. Adenovirus can cause a hemor-rhagic enteritis and melena in addition to hepatic disease [54,115]. Clostridial enterotoxemia has been reported in Falconiformes with hemmorhagic enteritis and hepatic necrosis also due to *Clostridium perfringens* type A/B and C [116]. Most affected birds had concurrent infections or disease.

Neoplasia

Neoplasia of the lower GI tract of raptors has been infrequently reported. Cases documented include a proventricular adenocarcinoma in a great horned owl [117], a cloacal squamous cell carcinoma of unknown species [59], a cloacal papilloma of an unspecified raptor [59], a malignant small intestinal lymphoma of an unspecified raptor [59], fibrosarcoma of the colon (numerous subcutaneous fibrosarcomas also found) in a red-tailed hawk [118], and lymphosarcoma of the colon in a mountain caracara (*Phalco-boenus megalopterus*) (E. Klaphake, personal communication, 2004).

Accessory organ diseases

Liver

Hepatic disease is common in raptors, and can be due to the numerous disease etiologies passing through the liver from the intestines or spread via a hematogenous route. Hepatic lipidosis was reported in a barred owl (*Strix varia*) with successful medical management [119]. Acute septicemic spiro-chetosis due to a *Borrelia sp.* in a northern spotted owl (*Strix occidentalis caurina*) caused mortality and hepatomegaly [120]. Avian tuberculosis has been reported in raptors to cause morbidity and mortality [121–124]. Tularemia was determined to be the cause of death in a rough-legged buzzard (*Buteo lagopus*) and an Ural owl (*Strix uralensis*) [125]. An attempt to induce toxoplasmosis in owls found no clinical signs from 40 to 70 days after exposure, however, Toxoplasma gondii was isolated from tissues and *T gondii* antibodies had developed in all owls [126]. Fatal cases of toxoplasmosis have been reported in a barred owl (*Strix varia*) and a bald eagle (*Haliaeetus leucocephalus*) [127,128]. Adenovirus have been seen or suspected in a variety of raptor species [54]. Birds surviving an adenovirus infection can become carriers, and the virus can persist in the environment [54,115].

Numerous herpesviruses have been identified in raptors, sometimes being called "inclusion body hepatitis" [129]. Three different raptor groups can be affected, leading to a description of falcon herpesvirus, owl herpesvirus, and eagle herpesvirus [129–135]. Owl and falcon herpesvirus are antigenically similar to each other and to pigeon herpesvirus, suggesting pigeons may be the source [54]. Herpesvirus infection creates tissue necrosis primarily in the liver, but pharyngeal lesions can also be found [129]. Acute death is often the initial sign with herpesvirus infection, although a period of anorexia, depression, and lethargy may preceed it. Species sensitivity to herpesvirus has been suggested, with gyrfalcons, prairie falcons of greatest concern [129]. Treatment with acyclovir at 80 mg/kg every 8 hours by mouth has been suggested in affected birds in addition to supportive care [54].

Adenoviruses have also been reported in raptors and are also referred to as "inclusion body hepatitis" [54,115]. Acute death from hepatitis is the classic presentation, with transmission oral from fecal or respiratory excretions. Vertical transmission has been reported [129].

Neoplasia of the liver of raptors has not been frequently reported. Cases include a hepatic fibrosarcoma in an unspecified raptor, hepatic adenocarcinoma (2) one as a metastasis in unspecified raptors, metastasized hepatic carcinoma in an unspecified raptor, bile duct carcinoma (3) in a red-tailed hawk, a golden eagle, and a northern goshawk, Marek's disease-induced hepatic tumors in a great horned owl, malignant hepatic lymphoma in an unspecified raptor, and hepatic lymphoid leucosis (4) in a merlin, a gray kestrel, a harris hawk, and an Eurasian eagle owl [54]. Cholangiocarcinoma has been reported in a red-tailed hawk [136] and metastatic cholangiocellular carcinoma in a golden eagle [137].

Pancreas

Only one raptor-specific report was found involving the pancreas, which was a case of pancreatic atrophy in a peregrine falcon [138]. No reports were found of pancreatic neoplasia in raptors. Steatorrhea characterized by brown sticky feces can be in an indication of pancreatic insufficiency and has been documented in raptors [19].

Summary

   Raptors are commonly presented to veterinarians by wildlife rehabilitatorsor falconers, and represent an important patient group. Understanding the variations in GI anatomy and physiology of these carnivorous birds from the more commonly seen psittacine birds is critical to the effective diagnosis and management of GI disease in raptors. The successful management of raptor GI patients hinge on an understanding of these diseases and their unique characteristics in raptors.

References

[1] Handrich Y, Nicolas L, Lemaho Y. Winter starvation in captive common barn owls—physiological states and reversible limits. Auk 1993;110:458–69.

[2] Sherrod SK. Diets of North American Falconiformes. J Raptor Res 1978;12(3/4):49–121.

[3] Johnsgard PA. Natural histories of individual species. In: Hawks, eagles, falcons of North America. Washington (DC): Smithsonian Institution; 1990. p. 97–328.

[4] Johnsgard PA. Natural histories of North American owls. In: North American owls—biology and natural history. Washington (DC): Smithsonian Institution; 1988. p. 93–238.

[5] Bose M, Guidali F. Seasonal and geographic differences in the diet of the barn owl in an agro-ecosystem in northern Italy. J Raptor Res 2001;35:240–6.

[6] Martinez JE, Calvo JF. Diet and breeding success of eagle owl in southeastern Spain: effect of rabbit haemorrhagic disease. J Raptor Res 2001;35:259–62.

[7] Vargas J, Landaeta C, Simonetti JA. Bats as prey of barn owls (*Tyto alba*) in a tropical savanna in Bolivia. J Raptor Res 2002;36:146–8.

[8] Tabaka CS, Ullrey DE, Sikarskie JG, et al. Diet, cast composition and energy and nutrient intake of red-tailed hawks (*Buteo jamaicensis*), great horned owls (*Bubo virginianus*), and turkey vultures (*Cathartes aura*). J Zoo Wildl Med 1996;27:187–96.

[9] Clum NJ, Fitzpatrick MP, Dierenfeld ES. Nutrient content of five species of domestic animals commonly fed to captive raptors. J Raptor Res 1997;31:267–72.

[10] Deem SL, Terrell SP, Forrester DJ. A retrospective study of morbidity and mortality of raptors in Florida: 1988–1994. J Zoo Wildl Med 1998;29:160–4.

[11] Ress S, Guyer C. A retrospective study of mortality and rehabilitation of raptors in the southeastern United States. J Raptor Res 2004;38:77–81.

[12] Franson JC, Thomas NJ, Smith MR, et al. A retrospective study of postmortem findings in red-tailed hawks. J Raptor Res 1996;30:7–14.

[13] Franson JC, Little SE. Diagnostic findings in 132 great horned owls. J Raptor Res 1996;30: 1–6.

[14] Work TM, Hale J. Causes of owl mortality in Hawaii, 1992 to 1994. J Wildl Dis 1996;32: 266–73.

[15] Wayland M, Wilson LK, Elliott JE, et al. Mortality, morbidity, and lead poisoning of eagles in western Canada, 1986–1998. J Raptor Res 2003;37:8–18.

[16] Klasing KC. Anatomy and physiology of the digestive system. In: Comparative avian nutrition. Oxon (UK): CAB International; 1998. p. 9–35.

[17] Barton NW, Houston DC. Factors influencing the size of some internal organs in raptors. J Raptor Res 1996;30:219–23.

[18] Denbow DM. Gastrointestinal anatomy and physiology. In: Whittow GC, editor. Sturkie's avian physiology. 5th edition. San Diego (CA): Academic Press; 2000. p. 299–321.

[19] Redig PT, Ackermann J. Raptors. In: Tully TN, Lawton MPC, Martin PC, Dorrestein GM, editors. Avian medicine. Oxford (UK): Butterworth-Heinemann; 2000. p. 180–214.

[20] Csermely D, Berte L, Camoni R. Prey killing by Eurasian kestrels: the role of the foot and the significance of bill and talons. J Avian Biol 1998;29:10–6.

[21] King AS, McLelland J. Birds: their structure and function. 2nd editon. Bath (UK): The Pitman Press; 1984. p. 84–109.

[22] Fox N. Structure and function. In: Understanding the bird of prey. Blaine (WA): Hancock House Publishers Ltd; 1995. p. 16–57.

[23] Nicholls MK, Love OP, Bird DM. An evaluation of methyl anthranilate, amino-acetophenone, and unfamiliar coloration as feeding repellents to American kestrels. J Raptor Res 2000;34:311–8.

[24] Lamberski N, Hull AC, Fish AM, et al. A survey of the choanal and cloacal aerobic bacterial flora in free-living and captive red-tailed hawks (*Buteo jamaicensis*) and cooper's hawks (*Accipiter cooperii*). J Avian Med Surg 2003;17:131–5.

[25] Morishita TY, Lowenstine LJ, Hirsh DC, et al. *Pateurella multocida* in raptors: prevalence and characterization. Avian Dis 1996;40:908–18.

[26] Zucca P. Anatomy. In: Cooper JE, editor. Birds of prey: health and disease. 3rd edition. Oxford (UK): Blackwell Science Ltd; 2002. p. 13–21.

[27] Macwhirter P. Basic anatomy, physiology and nutrition. In: Tully TN, Lawton MPC, Martin PC, Dorrestein GM, editors. Avian medicine. Oxford (UK): Butterworth-Heinemann; 2000. p. 1–25.

[28] Johnsgard PA. Foraging ecology and foods. In: Hawks, eagles, falcons of North America. Washington (DC): Smithsonian Institution; 1990. p. 23–38.

[29] Houston DC, Copsey JA. Bone digestion and intestinal morphology of the bearded vulture. J Raptor Res 1994;28:73–8.

[30] Yoram YT, Wool D. Do the contents of barn owl pellets accurately represent the proportion of prey species in the field? Condor 1997;99:972–6.

[31] Redpath SM, Clarke R, Madders M, et al. Assessing raptor diet: comparing pellets, prey remains, and observational data at hen harrier nests. Condor 2001;103:184–8.

[32] Akaki C, Duke GE. Egestion of chitin in pellets of American kestrels and eastern screech owls. J Raptor Res 1998;32:286–9.

[33] Clench MH, Mathias JR. Motility responses to fasting in the gastrointestinal-tract of 3 avian species. Condor 1995;97:1041–7.

[34] Duke GE, Reynhout J, Tereick AL, et al. Gastrointestinal morphology and motility in American kestrels receiving high or low fat diets. Condor 1997;99:123–31.

[35] Redig PT. Raptors. In: Altman RB, Clubb SL, Dorrenstein GM, Quesenberry K, editors. Avian medicine and surgery. Philadelphia (PA): WB Saunders; 1997. p. 918–28.

[36] Smith WA, Mazet JAK, Hirsh DC. *Salmonella* in California wildlife species: prevalence in rehabilitation centers and characterization of isolates. J Zoo Wildl Med 2002;33: 228–35.

[37] Battisti A, Guardo GD, Agrimi U, et al. Embryonic and neonatal mortality from salmonellosis in captive bred raptors. J Wildl Dis 1998;34:64–72.

[38] Oyarzabal OA, Conner DE, Hoerr FJ. Incidence of Campylobacters in the intestine of avian species in Alabama. Avian Dis 1995;39:147–51.

[39] Irokanulo EO, Makinde AA, Akuesgi CO, Ekwonu M. *Cryptococcus neoformans var neoformans* isolated from droppings of captive birds in Nigeria. J Wildl Dis 1997;33:343–5.

[40] Rupley AE. Gastrointestinal signs. In: Manual of avian practice. Philadelphia (PA): WB Saunders; 1997. p. 91–133.

[41] Heidenreich M. Diseases of specific organ systems. In: Birds of prey—medicine and management. Malden (MA): Blackwell Science Ltd; 1997. p. 168–218.

[42] Wheler CL. Orthopedic conditions of the avian head. Vet Clin North Am Exot Anim Pract 2002;5:83–95.

[43] Rosenfield RN, Bielefeldt J, Rosenfield LJ, et al. Prevalence of *Trichomonas gallinae* in nestling cooper's hawks among three North American populations. Wilson Bull 2002;114: 145–7.

[44] Boal CW, Mannan RW, Hudelson KS. Trichomoniasis in cooper's hawks from Arizona. J Wildl Dis 1998;34:590–3.

[45] Real J, Manosa S, Munoz E. Trichomoniasis in a Bonelli's eagle population in Spain. J Wildl Dis 2000;36:64–70.

[46] Ueblacker SN. Trichomoniasis in American kestrels (*Falco sparverius*) and eastern screech owls (*Otus asio*). In: Lumeij JT, Remple JD, Redig PT, Lierz m, Cooper JE, editors. Raptor biomedicine III. Lake Worth (FL): Zoological Education Network, Inc.; 2000. p. 59–64.

[47] Samour JH, Naldo JL. Diagnosis and therapeutic management of trichomoniasis in falcons in Saudi Arabia. J Avian Med Surg 2003;17:136–43.

[48] Samour JH, Bailey TA, Cooper JE. Trichomoniasis in birds of prey (Order Falconiformes) in Bahrain. Vet Rec 1995;136:358–62.

[49] Zucca P. Protozoa (Infectious diseases). In: Samour JH, editor. Avian medicine. Philadelphia (PA): Mosby; 2000. p. 225–31.

[50] Samour JH. Psuedomonas aeroginosa stomatitis as a sequela to trichomoniasis in captive Saker falcons (*Falco cherrug*). J Avian Med Surg 2000;14:113–7.

[51] Samour JH, Naldo JL. Diagnosis and therapeutic management of candidiasis in falcons in Saudi Arabia. J Avian Med Surg 2002;16:129–32.

[52] Santiago C, Mills PA, Kirkpatrick CE. Oral capillariasis in a red-tailed hawk-treatment with fenbendazole. J Am Vet Med Assoc 1985;187:1205–6.

[53] Ritchie BW. Poxviridae. In: Avian viruses: function and control. Lake Worth (FL): Wingers Publishing, Inc.; 1995. p. 285–311.

[54] Forbes NA, Simpson GN. A review of viruses affecting raptors. Vet Rec 1997;141:123–6.

[55] Wheeldon EB, Sedgwick CJ, Schultz TA. Epornitic of avian pox in a raptor rehabilitation center. J Am Vet Med Assoc 1985;187:1202–4.

[56] Samour JH, Cooper JE. Avian pox in birds of prey (Order Falconiformes) in Bahrain. Vet Rec 1993;132:343–5.

[57] Dutton CJ, Cooper JE, Allchurch AF. The pathology and diseases of the Mauritius kestrel (*Falco punctatus*). In: Lumeij JT, Remple JD, Redig PT, Lierz M, Cooper JE, editors. Raptor biomedicine III. Lake Worth (FL): Zoological Education Network, Inc.; 2000. p. 147–56.

[58] Scope A, Frey H. Diseases and mortality causes in captive and free-ranging bearded vultures (*Gypaetus barbatus*). In: Lumeij JT, Remple JD, Redig PT, Lierz M, Cooper JE, editors. Raptor biomedicine III. Lake Worth (FL): Zoological Education Network, Inc.; 2000. p. 157–62.

[59] Forbes NA, Cooper JE, Higgins RJ. Neoplasms of birds of prey. In: Lumeij JT, Remple JE, Redig PT, Lierz M, Cooper JE, editors. Raptor biomedicine III. Lake Worth (FL): Zoological Education Network, Inc.; 2000. p. 127–46.

[60] Morishita TY, Lowenstine LJ, Hirsh DC, et al. *Pasteurella multocida* in raptors: Prevalence and characterization. Avian Dis 1996;40:908–18.

[61] Jenkins J. Surgery of the avian reproductive and gastrointestinal systems. Vet Clin North Am Exot Anim Pract 2000;3:673–92.

[62] Tuggle BN, Schmeling SK. Parasites of the bald eagle (*Haliaeetus leucocephalus*) of North America. J Wildl Dis 1982;18:501–6.

[63] Lindsay DS, Ambrus SI, Blagburn BL. *Frenkelia* sp.-like infection in the small intestine of a red-tailed hawk. J Wildl Dis 1987;23:677–9.

[64] Hoberg EP, Cawthorn RJ, Hedstrom OR. Enteric coccidian (Apicomplexa) in the small intestine of the northern spotted owl (*Strix occidentalis caurina*). J Wildl Dis 1993;29:495–7.

[65] Kinsella JM, Foster GW, Forrester DJ. Parasitic helminthes of 6 species of hawks and falcons in Florida. J Raptor Res 1995;29:117–22.

[66] Averbeck GA, Cooney JD, Guarnera TR, et al. Exogenous stages of *Eimeria bemricki* n. sp. (Apicomplexa:Eimeriidae) from the great gray owl, *Strix nebulosa* (Foster). J Parasitol 1998;84:976–7.

[67] Volf J, Koudela B, Modry D. Two new species of Caryospora Leger, 1904 (Apicomplexa, Eimeriidae) from accipitrid raptors. Syst Parasitol 2000;46:23–7.

[68] Lacina D, Bird DM. Endoparasites of raptors—a review and update. In: Lumeij JT, Remple JD, Redig PT, Lierz M, Cooper JE, editors. Raptor biomedicine III. Lake Worth (FL): Zoological Education Network Inc.; 2000. p. 65–100.

[69] Krone O. Endoparasites in free-ranging birds of prey in Germany. In: Lumeij JT, Remple JD, Redig PT, Lierz M, Cooper JE, editors. Raptor biomedicine III. Lake Worth (FL): Zoological Education Network, Inc.; 2000. p. 101–16.

[70] Samour JH, Silvanose C. Parasitological findings in captive falcons in the United Arab Emirates. In: Lumeij JT, Remple JD, Redig PT, Lierz M, Cooper JE, editors. Raptor biomedicine III. Lake Worth (FL): Zoological Education Network, Inc.; 2000. p. 117–26.

[71] Papazahariadou MG, Georgiades GK, Komnenou ATH, et al. Caryospora species in a snowy owl (Nyctea scandiaca). Vet Rec 2001;148:54–5.

[72] Nakamura K, Ohyama T, Saito A, et al. Gizzard nematodiasis in Japanese mountain hawk eagle (Spizaetus nipalensis). Avian Dis 2001;45:751–4.

[73] Lierz M. Evaluation of the dosage of ivermectin in falcons. Vet Rec 2001;148:596–600.

[74] Forbes NA, Simpson GN. A review of viruses affecting raptors. Vet Rec 1997;141:123–6.

[75] Manvell RJ, Wernery U, Alexander DJ, et al. Newcastle disease (avian PMV-1) viruses in raptors. In: Lumeij JT, Remple JD, Redig PT, Lierz M, Cooper JE, editors. Raptor biomedicine III. Lake Worth (FL): Zoological Education Network, Inc.; 2000. p. 3–8.

[76] Schettler E, Langgenmach T, Sommer P, et al. Seroepizootiology of selected infectious disease agents in free-living birds of prey in Germany. J Wildl Dis 2001;37:145–52.

[77] Schettler E, Fickel J, Hotzel H, et al. Newcastle disease virus and Chlamydia psittaci in free-living raptors from eastern Germany. J Wildl Dis 2003;39:57–63.

[78] Toro H, Pavez EF, Gough RE, et al. Serum chemistry and antibody status to some avian pathogens of free-living and captive condors (Vultur gryphus) of central Chile. Avian Pathol 1997;26:339–45.

[79] Lublin A, Mechani S, Siman-Tov Y, et al. Sudden death of a bearded vulture (Gypaetus barbatus) possibly caused by Newcastle disease virus. Avian Dis 2001;45:741–4.

[80] Bonar CJ, Lewandowski AH, Schaul J. Suspected fenbendazole toxicosis in 2 vulture species (Gyps africanus, Torgos tracheliotus) and marabou storks (Leptoptilos crumeniferus). J Avian Med Surg 2003;17:16–9.

[81] Harrenstien LA, Tell LA, Vulliet R, et al. Disposition of enrofloxacin in red-tailed hawks (Buteo jamaicensis) and great horned owls (Bubo virginianus) after a single oral, intramuscular, or intravenous dose. J Avian Med Surg 2000;14:228–36.

[82] Oaks JL, Gilbert M, Virani MZ, et al. Diclofenac residues as the cause of vulture population decline in Pakistan. Nature 2004;427:630–3.

[83] Mateo R, Molina R, Grifols J, et al. Lead poisoning in a free ranging griffon vulture (Gyps fulvus). Vet Rec 1997;140:47–8.

[84] Kramer JL, Redig PT. Sixteen years of lead poisoning in eagles, 1980–95: an epizootiologic view. J Raptor Res 1997;31:327–32.

[85] Miller MJR, Restani M, Harmata AR, et al. A comparison of blood lead levels in bald eagles from two regions on the Great Plains of North America. J Wildl Dis 1998;34:704–14.

[86] Saito K, Kurosawa N, Shimura R. Lead poisoning in endangered sea-eagles (Haliaeetus albicilla, H. pelagicus) in eastern Hokkaido through ingestion of shot sika deer (Cervus nipon). In: Lumeij JT, Remple JD, Redig PT, Lierz M, Cooper JE, editors. Raptor biomedicine III. Lake Worth (FL): Zoological Education Network, Inc.; 2000. p. 163–8.

[87] Miller MJR, Wayland AE, Dzus EH, et al. Availability and ingestion of lead shotshell pellets by migrant bald eagles in Saskatchewan. J Raptor Res 2000;34:167–74.

[88] Miller MJR, Wayland ME, Bortolotti GR. Hemograms for and nutritional condition of migrant bald eagles tested for exposure to lead. J Wildl Dis 2001;37:481–8.

[89] Samour JH, Naldo J. Diagnosis and therapeutic management of lead toxicosis in falcons in Saudi Arabia. J Avian Med Surg 2002;16:16–20.

[90] McBride TJ, Smith JP, Gross HP, et al. Blood-lead and ALAD activity levels of cooper's hawks (*Aciipiter cooperii*) migrating through the southern Rocky Mountains. J Raptor Res 2004;38:118–24.

[91] DeMent SH, Chisolm JJ, Barber JC, et al. Lead exposure in an "Urban" peregrine falcon and its avian prey. J Wildl Dis 1986;22:238–44.

[92] Chandler RB, Strong AM, Kaufman CC. Elevated lead levels in urban house sparrows: a threat to sharp-shinned hawks and merlins? J Raptor Res 2004;38:62–8.

[93] Carpenter JW, Pattee OH, Fritts SH, et al. Experimental lead poisoning in turkey vultures (*Cathartes aura*). J Wildl Dis 2003;39:96–104.

[94] Platt SR, Helmick KE, Graham J, et al. Peripheral neuropathy in a turkey vulture with lead toxicosis. J Am Vet Med Assoc 1999;214:1218–20.

[95] Jagoe CH, Bryan AL, Brant HA, et al. Mercury in bald eagle nestlings from South Carolina, USA. J Wildl Dis 2002;38:706–12.

[96] Stout JH, Trust KA. Elemental and organchlorine residues in bald eagles from Adak Island, Alaska. J Wildl Dis 2002;38:511–7.

[97] Stone WB, Okoniewski JC, Stedlin JR. Poisoning of wildlife with anticoagulant rodenticides in New York. J Wildl Dis 1999;35:187–93.

[98] Wheeldon EB, Bogan JA, Taylor DJ. Dieldrin poisoning in a captive bird of prey. Vet Rec 1975;97:412.

[99] Franson JC, Kolbe EJ, Carpenter JW. Famphur toxicosis in a bald eagle. J Wildl Dis 1985; 21:318–20.

[100] Wiemeyer SN, Hills EF, Carpenter JW, et al. Acute oral toxicity of sodium cyanide in birds. J Wildl Dis 1986;22:538–46.

[101] Blus LJ. Effects of pesticides on owls in North America. J Raptor Res 1996;30:198–206.

[102] Allen GT, Veatch JK, Stroud RK, et al. Winter poisoning of coyotes and raptors with furadan-laced carcass baits. J Wildl Dis 1996;32:385–9.

[103] Elliott JE, Langelier KM, Mineau P, et al. Poisoning of bald eagles and red-tailed hawks by carbofuran and fensulfothion in the Fraser Delta of British Columbia. J Wildl Dis 1996;32: 486–91.

[104] Wood PB, Viverette C, Goodrich L, et al. Environmental contaminant levels in sharp-shinned hawks from the eastern United States. J Raptor Res 1996;30:136–44.

[105] Garcelon DK, Thomas NJ. DDE poisoning in an adult bald eagle. J Wildl Dis 1997;33: 299–303.

[106] Henny CJ, Galushin VM, Dudin PI, et al. Organochlorine pesticides, PCBs, and mercury in hawk, falcon, eagle, and owl eggs from the Lipetsk, Voronezh, Novgorod, and Saratov regions, Russia, 1992–1993. J Raptor Res 1998;32:143–50.

[107] Keith JO, Bruggers RL. Review of hazards to raptors from pest control in Sahelian Africa. J Raptor Res 1998;32:151–8.

[108] Frank RA, Lutz RS. Productivity and survival of great horned owls exposed to dieldrin. Condor 1999;101:331–9.

[109] Mineau P, Fletcher MR, Glaser LC, et al. Poisoning of raptors with organophosphorus and carbamate pesticides with emphasis on Canada, US, and UK. J Raptor Res 1999;33:1–37.

[110] Ostrowski S, Shobrak M. Pesticide poisoning in a free-ranging lappet-faced vulture (*Torgos tracheliotus*). Vet Rec 2001;149:396–7.

[111] Wobeser G, Bollinger T, Leighton FA, et al. Secondary poisonings of eagles following intentional poisoning of coyotes with anticholinesterase pesticides in western Canada. J Wildl Dis 2004;40:163–72.

[112] Woodley SJ, Meyer KD, Kirk DA, Pearce PA. Contaminant levels, eggshell thinning, and productivity in sharp-shinned hawks in Fundy National Park, New Brunswick. J Raptor Res 2004;38:69–77.

[113] Mobley JA, Stidham TA. Great horned owl death from predation of a toxic California newt. Wilson Bull 2000;112:563–4.

[114] Murnane RD, Meerdink G, Rideout BA, et al. Ethylene glycol toxicosis in a captive-bred released Califronia condor (*Gymnogyps californianus*). J Zoo Wildl Med 1995;26:306–10.

[115] Ritchie BW. Adenoviridae. In: Avian viruses: function and control. Lake Worth (FL): Wingers Publishing, Inc.; 1995. p. 313–33.

[116] Wernery U, Kinne J, Sharma A, et al. Clostrium enterotoxaemia in Flaconiformes in the United Arab Emirates. In: Lumeij JT, Remple JD, Redig PT, Lierz M, Cooper JE, editors. Raptor biomedicine III. Lake Worth (FL): Zoological Education Network, Inc.; 2000. p. 35–51.

[117] Yonemaru K, Sakai H, Asaoka Y, et al. Proventricular adenocarcinoma in a Humboldt penguin (*Spheniscus humboldti*) and a great horned owl (*Bubo virginianus*); identification of origin by mucin histochemistry. Avian Pathol 2004;33:77–81.

[118] Stetter MD, Nichols DK. Multiple mesenchymal neoplasms in a young red-tailed hawk (*Buteo jamicensis*). J Zoo Wildl Med 1993;24:68–72.

[119] James SB, Raphael BL, Clippinger T. Diagnosis and treatment of hepatic lipidosis in a barred owl (*Strix varia*). J Avian Med Surg 2000;14:268–72.

[120] Thomas NJ, Bunikis J, Barbour AG, et al. Fatal spirochetosis due to a relapsing fever-like *Borerelia* sp. in a northern spotted owl. J Wildl Dis 2002;38:187–93.

[121] Bucke D, Mawdesley-Thomas E. Tuberculosis in a barn owl (*Tyto alba*). Vet Rec 1974;95: 373.

[122] Mollhoff WJ. Avian tuberculosis in a saw-whet owl. Wilson Bull 1976;88:505.

[123] Sykes GP. Tuberculosis in a red-tailed hawk (*Buteo jamaicensis*). J Wildl Dis 1982;18:495–9.

[124] Tell LA, Ferrell ST, Gibbons PM. Avian mycobacteriosis in free-living raptors in California: 6 cases (1997–2001). J Avian Med Surg 2004;18:30–40.

[125] Morner T, Mattsson R. Tularemia in a rough-legged buzzard (*Buteo lagopus*) and a Ural owl (*Strix uralensis*). J Wildl Dis 1983;19:360–1.

[126] Dubey JP, Porter SL, Tseng F, et al. Induced toxoplasmosis in owls. J Zoo Wildl Med 1992; 23:98–102.

[127] Mikaelian I, Dubey JP, Martineau D. Severe hepatitis resulting from toxoplasmosis in a barred owl (*Strix varia*) from Quebec, Canada. Avian Dis 1997;41:738–40.

[128] Szabo KA, Mense MG, Lipscomb TP, et al. Fatal toxoplasmosis in a bald eagle (*Haliaeetus leucocephalus*). J Parasitol 2004;90:907–8.

[129] Ritchie BW. Herpesviridae. In: Avian viruses: function and control. Lake Worth (FL): Wingers Publishing, Inc.; 1995. p. 171–222.

[130] Aini I, Shih LM, Castro AE, et al. Comparison of herpesvirus isolates from falcons, pigeons, and psittacines by restriction endonuclease analysis. J Wildl Dis 1993;29:196–202.

[131] Gough RE, Drury SEN, George AD, et al. Isolation and identification of a falcon herpesvirus. Vet Rec 1993;132:220–1.

[132] Mozos E, Hervas J, Moyano T, et al. Inclusion-body disease in a peregrine falcon (*Falco peregrinus*)—histological and ultrastructural study. Avian Pathol 1994;23:175–81.

[133] Ramis A, Majo N, Pumarola M, et al. Herpesvirus hepatitis in two eagles in Spain. Avian Dis 1994;38:197–200.

[134] Gough RE, Drury SEN, Higgins RJ, et al. Isolation of a herpesvirus from a snowy owl (*Nyctea scandiaca*). Vet Rec 1995;136:541–2.

[135] Gough RE, Capau I, Wernery U. Herpesvirus infections in raptors. In: Lumeij JT, Remple JD, Redig PT, Lierz M, Cooper JE, editors. Raptor biomedicine III. Lake Worth (FL): Zoological Education Network, Inc.; 2000. p. 9–12.

[136] Hartup BK, Steinberg H, Forrest LJ. Cholangiocarcinoma in a red-tailed hawk (*Buteo jamaicensis*). J Zoo Wildl Med 1996;27:539–43.

[137] Mikaelian I, Patenaude R, Girard C, et al. Metastatic cholangiocellular carcinoma and renal adenocarcinoma in a golden eagle (*Aquila chrysaetos*). Avian Pathol 1998;27:321–5.

[138] Samour JH, Naldo JL. Pancreatic atrophy in a peregrine falcon (*Falco peregrinus*). Vet Rec 2002;151:124.

ELSEVIER
SAUNDERS

VETERINARY
CLINICS
Exotic Animal Practice

Vet Clin Exot Anim 8 (2005) 329–349

Disorders of the Psittacine Gastrointestinal Tract

Tarah L. Hadley, DVM

The University of Tennessee, College of Veterinary Medicine, Department of Small Animal Clinical Sciences, Knoxville, TN 37996-4544, USA

The gastrointestinal (GI) tract is one of the most complicated organ systems in birds. The complexity of this organ system is underscored by knowledge that diseases affecting other organ systems in the body tend to impact the function of the GI tract. This review highlights some of the major GI diseases (infectious, neoplastic, toxic, and traumatic) that affect psittacine bird species.

Anatomy and physiology of the avian gastrointestinal tract

Oropharynx

In birds, the oropharynx is comprised of the oral cavity and the pharynx [1]. Unlike mammals, there is no distinct division between the two regions [1]. It is lined by stratified squamous epithelium [2]. In place of a soft palate, birds have a median longitudinal fissure called a choana, which links the oral cavity to the nasal cavity [1]. The surface of the oropharynx, including the edge of the choana, is lined by numerous papillae [2]. The palate of most birds has numerous ridges located rostral and lateral to the choana that aid in the removal of seed shells [2]. The infundibular cleft lies caudal to the choana and serves as an opening to the auditory tubes [1].

The tongue of psittacine species is used to manipulate food in the oral cavity and does not protrude beyond the beak opening [2]. The psittacine tongue may be darkly pigmented. It is short, thick, and fleshy due to intrinsic muscles and adapted for manipulating seeds and nuts [2]. The caudal portion of the tongue contains caudally directed papilla called the laryngeal mound. The laryngeal mound helps to move food boluses toward

E-mail address: TLHADLEY@utk.edu

the back of the oral cavity during swallowing and to prevent regurgitation [1,2]. Salivary glands may be found in multiple locations along the roof and floor of the mouth [2]. They tend to be well developed in some bird species, such as seed eaters, whose diet consists primarily of dry material [2]. Mucous secreted by the salivary glands lubricates food and permits greater ease of swallowing. The salivary glands of some birds may also secrete amylase, which aids with carbohydrate digestion [1].

Esophagus and crop

The esophagus of birds is thin-walled and highly distensible with a relative diameter that is greater than the esophagus of mammals [1,2]. Its longitudinal folds are lined by incompletely keratinized stratified squamous epithelium with numerous mucous glands [1,2]. Contrary to mammals, the avian esophagus lies along the right side of the cervix [2]. Salivary glands in the esophagus primarily secrete mucous [1]. The crop is located immediately cranial to the thoracic inlet at the termination of the esophagus. In many psittacine species, the crop is very large and may distend into a saclike diverticulum that extends from one side of the neck to the other [2]. Like the esophagus, the crop is also lined with incompletely keratinized stratified squamous epithelium [1]. Mild carbohydrate digestion by the enzyme amylase may occur in the region of the crop [1].

Stomach

In birds, the stomach consists of two separate portions: the glandular proventriculus and the muscular ventriculus. The proventriculus is the avian equivalent of the mammalian stomach [1]. The proventriculus connects to the crop and is the most cranial portion. No distinct boundary exists between the proventriculus and the crop except that in non–meat-eaters, the proventriculus lacks the longitudinal folds of the esophagus [2]. Its size and shape varies among bird species, but it is generally characterized by a fusiform shape [1]. The luminal surface of the proventriculus is lined by papilla that serve as openings for gastric glands [1,2]. The gastric glands are either unilobular or multilobular and consist of tall columnar cells that secrete mucous during feeding [2]. These cells, called oxynticopeptic cells, also secrete hydrochloric acid and pepsin [1,2]. This is different from mammals, where each of these substances is produced by two separate cell types [2]. The oxynticopeptic cells project into the proventricular lumen and give the mucosal surface a serrated appearance [2].

The ventriculus, commonly referred to as the gizzard, follows the proventriculus. An intermediate zone separates the two stomach compartments [1,2]. The ventriculus aids in mechanical digestion or crushing of food items [1,2]. The type of diet ingested by the bird dictates the gross appearance and structure of the ventriculus [2]. In granivores, for instance, the ventriculus is thick walled and well developed to accommodate food items that might otherwise be indigestible [2]. Frugivores tend to have a small ventriculus that terminates in an band-like structure or vestigial diverticulum [2]. Function of the ventriculus is facilitated by the oppositional movement of thick and thin pairs of muscles in an environment of extremely high pressures and powerful contractions [1,2]. Once food items are crushed, they are more susceptible to the effects of proteolytic enzymes and acids in the stomach [2].

A cuticle or koilin layer consisting of a carbohydrate–protein complex lines the inside of the highly muscular portion of the ventriculus [1,2]. The koilin layer protects the stomach chamber from injury during the mechanical breakdown of hard food and from the effects of acid and proteolytic enzymes [1,2]. Due to the reflux of duodenal bile pigments, the koilin may appear green, brown, or even yellow in color [2]. In most birds, the koilin is continually produced by mucous glands as it is worn away [1]. Other birds will slough the koilin layer in its entirety [1]. The pylorus marks the termination of the ventriculus and the start of the duodenum. Its function is largely unknown [1,2]. One theory suggests that the pylorus may slow down the movement of hard particles before entry into the duodenum [1].

The motility of the avian stomach differs from the mammalian stomach [1]. In birds, the movement of food items occurs in three phases. During the first phase, the isthmus, or intermediate zone region, closes [1]. The thin muscles of the ventriculus contract and the pylorus relaxes, allowing food materials to be pushed into the duodenum [1]. In the second phase of motility, the isthmus relaxes while the duodenum and thick muscles of the ventriculus contract, refluxing food items back into the proventriculus [1]. The contraction of the proventriculus is the third and final phase which completes the motility cycle [1]. The nerve plexus located at the isthmus is considered to be the pacemaker of the GI motility cycle [1].

Small intestine

The small intestine is the primary site for chemical digestion and food absorption [2]. Similar to mammals, the small intestine of birds is divided into the duodenum, jejunum, and the ileum, but these three areas of the GI tract may not always be distinguishable either grossly or histologically [1]. The duodenum is typically U-shaped, and has a proximal descending portion as well as a distal ascending portion that are held together by mesentery [2]. Bile and pancreatic ducts in most birds are located close together at the most distal portion of the ascending duodenal loop [2]. Bile, which is produced and secreted by the liver, is responsible for emulsifying lipids so they are more easily digested by enzymes [1]. The avian exocrine pancreas secretes many digestive enzymes that are similar to those secreted by mammalian species [2]. During postmortem examination, the duodenum is easily identified as the most ventral bowel loop [2].

The jejunum and ileum also form U-shaped loops, but they typically have a narrower diameter [2]. The latter two small intestinal segments are separated by the vitelline diverticulum—also known as Meckel's diverticulum—which is a short remnant of the yolk sac [1,2]. The total intestinal length will vary among bird species depending on the diet. Frugivores tend to have a shorter intestinal length compared with granivores [1]. Histologically, the intestines are made of four layers. The innermost layer is the mucosal layer followed by the submucosal, muscular tunic, and serosal layers. Villi are present but lack central lacteals [1]. The villous epithelium, however, does contain goblet, chief, and endocrine cells [1].

Large intestine and cloaca

In many birds, including granivores, paired ceca arise near the junction of the ileum with the rectum [1,2]. In psittacine species, ceca may be reduced in size or number or absent altogether [1,2]. The morphology of the ileocecal junction only permits liquid or very small particles to gain entrance to the ceca [1]. Overall, the motility of the ceca is not well understood [1].

The rectum in birds is a short tube-like structure that consists of numerous villi and a few goblet cells unlike mammals, which have more goblet cells and less villi [1]. Rectal motility is continuous and occurs in antiperistaltic waves [1]. Rectal antiperistalsis is primarily responsible for moving urine from the urodeum into the colon and ceca [1]. The only time antiperistalsis of the colon is interrupted is just before defecation, when strong contractions in the proximal colon move contents aborally until defecation occurs a few seconds later [1].

The cloaca serves as a common waste compartment for three chambers [1]. The coprodeum is the cranial-most chamber into which excreta from the rectum empties [1]. Contrast studies in healthy psittacine birds show it takes as long as 4 hours for barium sulfate to reach and fill the cloaca from the time of ingestion [3]. The remaining chambers, the urodeum and proctodeum, serve other excretory functions. Although the rectum and cloaca play key roles in the reabsorption of water, water is primarily absorbed from the small and large intestines and ceca [1].

The paired ceca vary in size [4]. Large ceca are typically associated with herbivores and granivores [4]. NaCl and water are absorbed by the ceca while potassium is secreted [4]. Large amounts of intestinal and ureteral water and solutes move together with small-sized solids into the ceca by peristalsis and antiperistalsis in the ileum and colon, respectively [4]. Cecal function studies show inflow rates of about 20% each from ureteral urine and oral ingestion [4].

In most birds, urine from the ureters flows backward by retrograde peristalsis from the urodeum into the coprodeum and colon [4]. This permits the absorptive epithelia of the lower gut to come into contact with a mixture of urine and chyme from the ileum [4]. The coprodeum and colon have columnar epithelial cells that permit absorption or secretion of ions and water [4]. Some of the urine and chyme will enter the paired ceca [4]. In addition to ions and water, nutrients such as short-chain fatty acids are absorbed here [4]. Urinary refluxing may serve a variety of functions, including reclamation of water, electrolytes, nitrogen, or energy that would be otherwise lost [4].

Although coprodeum and colon serve as a common storage chamber for ureteral urine and chyme, they have differing transport properties [4]. Coprodeum and colon are heavily influenced by sodium chloride (NaCl) intake [4]. The rate of Na absorption is activated by NaCl depletion and suppressed by NaCl loading [4]. The secretion of hydrogen leads to an acid microclimate on the mucosal surface of the coprodeum and colon [4]. The acid microclimate aids in colonic absorption of short-chain fatty acids, especially propionate [4]. Overall, the colon functions as the workhorse for recovery of salt and water from ureteral urine and chyme, whereas the coprodeum functions to fine tune total excretion [4].

Disorders of the psittacine gastrointestinal tract

Oropharynx

Avian poxvirus infection

Avian poxvirus, or avipoxvirus, is a large DNA virus of the Poxviridae family. When this virus infects avian species it forms characteristic intracytoplasmic inclusion bodies called Bollinger bodies in the epithelial cells of the oral cavity [5]. The virus may be transmitted from birds that are latently infected or via biting arthropods in the environment, such as mosquitoes [5]. Because mosquitoes tend to be the predominant vector for the virus, the most common time for infection occurs in the late summer or fall when mosquito populations are at their highest [5]. Mosquitoes that acquire avipoxvirus from an infected bird may harbor the virus in their salivary glands for as long as 8 weeks [5]. Direct transmission of the virus occurs through damaged epithelium [5]. Infection is usually subacute, and once infected, it may take a bird 3 to 4 weeks to recover from the infection [5].

In psittacine bird species, the diphtheroid or "wet form" is the most predominant form of avipoxvirus that occurs [5]. Typically, clinical signs are affected by the location of lesions [6]. Clinical signs in these birds may include fibrinous yellow-white plaques attached to the mucosa of the tongue, pharynx, and larynx that are usually difficult to remove [5,7]. Sometimes these lesions may coalesce into a larger lesion and prevent birds from swallowing food [5,6]. Another complication may cause dyspnea, complete occlusion of the glottis, or excessive bleeding if disrupted [5,6]. Definitive diagnosis of avipoxvirus may be achieved with demonstration of Bollinger bodies in biopsy samples [5].

Recovery from disease may grant immunity of as long as 8 months from future infection but immunity may be of shorter duration [5]. Vaccination with inactivated psittacine poxvirus in the healthy bird may provide some protection from avipoxvirus infections and may be recommended in high-risk populations, such as imported birds, birds exposed to imported birds, or birds with a high level of exposure to mosquito populations [5,6]. A preventative plan is needed, as poxviruses are extremely hardy and transmission may occur with direct contact with an infected bird as well as fomites [6]. Treatment of infected birds with acyclovir has been recommended, but there is no data to support its efficacy [7].

Hypovitaminosis A

A vitamin A deficiency may occur in birds that are predominantly fed seed-based diets [7]. On histopathology, vitamin A deficiency is character-ized by squamous metaplasia of the salivary glands of the oral cavity [7,8]. A common clinical presentation includes blunting of the choanal papilla and white plaques on the mucous membranes of the oral cavity that are easily removed [9]. Diagnosis is usually presumptive based upon the diet. Treatment of hypovitaminosis A is usually with parenteral vitamin A (20,000 IU/kg intramuscularly) [7,10]. A recent study in cockatiels, however, suggests that these birds may actually be more sensitive to diets that contain excessive rather than deficient amounts of vitamin A [11]. Some birds that received diets high in vitamin A exhibited intensified vocalization patterns and developed pancreatitis compared with birds supplemented with less vitamin A [11].

Trauma

The oral cavity of psittacine bird species may be exposed to trauma from a variety of causes, including electrocution from biting electric cords, mate trauma, the ingestion of hot foods, or caustic and toxic materials [12]. A bird with trauma to the oral cavity may show signs of rubbing at its beak, difficulty prehending food or swallowing, gaping of the mouth, or yawning [12]. Tongue lacerations may require suturing due to the tendency to bleed profusely [12].

Psittacine birds have a propensity for chewing on toys, perches, and other items in their environment. A foreign body may become lodged in the oral cavity and cause lacerations of the tongue or mucous membranes, inability to prehend food, or problems with swallowing or breathing [7,13]. Oropharyn-geal foreign bodies may be diagnosed during a physical examination that includes a thorough inspection of the oral cavity with a bright light source. Radiographs of the skull may also provide evidence of foreign bodies that are not immediately visible. Removal of foreign bodies, which may need to take place under general anesthesia for ease of access to the oral cavity and decreased stress for the avian patient, is the recommended treatment. Punctures to mucous membranes may cause granulomas or abscesses and need to be debrided and treated with systemic broad-spectrum antibiotic medications.

Candidiasis

Infection of the oropharynx with *Candida albicans* is characterized by the formation of white plaques on the mucous membranes [12]. Among psittacine birds, young birds are the most susceptible to infection with this fungus secondary to crop stasis or other concurrent illness causing immunosuppression [12]. Adult birds may also become predisposed to infection due to concurrent illness, malnutrition, and prolonged antibiotic therapy [12].

Diagnosis of a yeast infection may be achieved with cytology of oral lesions [12]. A specific diagnosis may be obtained with a fungal culture [12]. Lesions are typically difficult to remove from the mucous membranes [12]. It is not possible to diagnose from gross appearance of the lesion alone. Treatment of *Candida* infections is usually with oral antifungal medications. The drugs most commonly used to treat local infection include nystatin (300,000 IU/kg by mouth every 12 hours for 7 to 14 days) and amphotericin B (0.25–1.0 mL by mouth every 24 hours for 4–5 days) [10]. Both drugs require contact with lesions to be effective [12]. Other antifungal medications like drugs from the azole family may be indicated in the event of systemic mycotic infections [10]. Diagnosis and treatment of concurrent illness may be of paramount importance to the improvement of the patient.

Neoplasia

Oropharyngeal neoplasms previously diagnosed in psittacine birds include fibrosarcoma, lymphosarcoma, and squamous cell carcinoma [12]. Biopsy of a lesion for histopathology provides a definitive diagnosis. Treatment options depend upon the neoplasm diagnosed. Complete surgical excision may be curative but may not always be possible. Other therapeutic options include chemotherapy or radiation therapy. Prognosis for malignant neoplasms is usually guarded to poor.

Papillomatosis

Papillomatosis, which may occur in the oral cavity as well as the rest of the GI tract, is commonly seen in macaws and other South American parrots [12]. This disease will be discussed in more detail under diseases of the cloaca.

Esophagus and crop

Esophageal/crop stasis

Decreased motility or stasis of the esophagus and crop is a syndrome that can occur in psittacine birds of all ages due to a variety of causes. Potential differentials for crop stasis include yeast overgrowth, crop atony or overstretching, heavy metal toxicosis, foreign body or food impaction, parasitism, inflammation of the esophagus or crop, an enlarged thyroid gland, or neuropathic gastric dilatation [7,14]. Young birds may be more susceptible to crop stasis secondary to yeast overgrowth during improper husbandry, such as the hand-feeding formula given in inappropriate amounts or at an inappropriate temperature. Adult birds with yeast overgrowth tend to have some other underlying illness that makes them less capable of fighting a fungal infection.

Diagnosis of crop stasis starts with a complete physical examination. The crop is located at the base of the keel region closer to the right side of the bird. A distended crop may sometimes be visible [12]. Another technique involves soaking the feathers in that area with saline or alcohol and using a bright light source to illuminate that area for better visualization [12]. Palpation of the crop may reveal distention with fluid or food material, or a combination of both. Care must be taken to palpate gently as birds have been known to regurgitate, leading to potential aspiration during handling. A complete history on the patient may provide some clues as to the cause of the stasis. The history may also direct the specific diagnostics that are performed in each case. Stained cytology of the crop contents or feces may provide evidence of budding yeasts.

Crop contents that are unable to move through to the proventriculus and ventriculus may acquire a sour odor over time. The contents may serve as a prime source of bacteria and the toxins they produce [15]. Removal of these contents is necessary to stabilize the patient [15,16]. A metal ball-tipped gavage tube or flexible red rubber catheter may be used to aspirate crop contents [15]. When the crop contents are doughy or difficult to aspirate, a small amount of a warm balanced electrolyte solution may be inserted via gavage, mixed with gentle palpation, and then aspirated. Birds with crop stasis, especially for long periods of time, usually require supportive care with a warm incubator and parenteral fluids to correct dehydration or metabolic imbalances. Use of systemic antibiotic, antifungal, or motility medications should be considered on a case-by-case basis.

Crop impaction

In young psittacine birds, impaction of the crop may occur secondary to inappropriate husbandry such as improper hand feeding amount or consistency or ingestion of bedding material by the chick [12]. Hand-feeding formulas prepared with inadequate amounts of water may "dry out" in the crop. As the liquid portion passes through the rest of the GI tract, the remaining dry material can continue to sit in the crop [12]. This material can become a substrate for bacterial and yeast overgrowth. When overgrowth of infectious agents occurs, the bird becomes prone to the development of dehydration, metabolic imbalances, and systemic disease [12].

A stained cytology of the feces or crop material may provide adequate evidence of infection and a basis to treat the infection. A culture and sensitivity of crop contents may also be warranted in cases of severe disease [12]. Treatment will depend on the condition of the patient but may include a warm water crop lavage and aspiration of crop contents. Parenteral fluids, a warm environment, or systemic antibiotic or antifungal medications may be needed for supportive care. Other considerations for impaction in young birds include foreign bodies, such as toys, grit, or cage substrate made of wood shavings or corn cob [7,12]. Differentials for crop impaction in adult birds are similar to those discussed in the section on crop stasis.

Foreign bodies

Unweaned and juvenile psittacine birds may be prone to ingestion of foreign bodies due to their inquisitive natures [7,17,18]. Examples of common foreign material ingested include cage substrate, grit, or toys. In adult psittacine birds, foreign body impactions may be secondary to ingluvioliths, excess grit ingestion, heavy metal ingestion, or ingestion of large food items that are difficult to pass beyond the level of the crop [7,16]. Clinical signs in birds with foreign bodies range from vomiting, regurgitation, decreased fecal production, anorexia, lethargy, and weight loss.

Diagnosis of crop foreign bodies may be obtained on palpation during a physical examination, and may require survey radiographs or radiographs with contrast media for diagnosis. Treatment may require endoscopic retrieval or ingluviotomy [19]. The viability of the crop should be assessed during endoscopy or surgery in case a partial crop resection needs to be performed. Another removal technique involves placing the head in a dependent position and flushing the foreign material out of the crop using a metal gavage tube or a soft red rubber catheter [18]. Intubation is re-commended during this procedure to prevent aspiration.

Some foreign objects may be manipulated from the crop to the oral cavity without sedation in very young birds [19]. Supportive care with a warm incubator, parenteral fluids, or systemic antibiotic or antifungal medications may be needed. If the foreign body advances to the level of the ventriculus or distal GI tract a celiotomy may be required for access to that portion of the GI tract.

Esophageal/crop lacerations and fistulas

Unweaned psittacine birds gavaged hand-feeding formula that is too hot may have thermal injury of the esophagus and crop as the formula makes its way through the upper GI tract. The damage to the crop may interfere with crop motility and result in crop stasis [12]. Mild burns cause temporary inflammation and edema of the tissue and may eventually resolve [12].

If the crop mucosa becomes traumatized and damaged by the extreme heat, a fistula develops in the crop [7,12]. Food left over in the crop or newly eaten food may leak out the fistula into the subcutaneous space. A similar injury may develop in the skin overlying the crop defect creating a full thickness fistula from the crop to the outside of the body. Some patients, especially those in the process of being weaned, present with a history of a voracious appetite with concurrent weight loss. On physical examination, the separation of moistened feathers in the area of the crop may reveal a hole in the tissue. Sometimes food contents may be visualized on the feathers of the pectoral area. Severe subcutaneous edema often develops in association with subcutaneous leakage of food material. This condition constitutes an emergency and surgical repair of the crop fistula should be performed as soon as possible.

Full-thickness fistulas to the outside of the body may require a waiting period of 3 to 5 days from presentation may be needed to give the tissue time to present itself as damaged. This will also allow time for the patient's condition to stabilize. Surgery performed too soon may result in failure of the repair. In the days before surgery, the area should be evacuated of feathers and flushed with a warm balanced electrolyte solution. A "crop bra" may be applied to the fistula using a light bandage in the shape of an X that wraps around the front of the bird. The "crop bra" allows the bird to eat and prevents food material from coming out of the fistula. The defect should be cleaned and the "crop bra" changed at least once daily. Some late stage crop fistulas may form a scab over the affected area [12].

Surgical repair involves removal of dead or necrotic tissue. Care must be taken to separate the crop from the overlying skin. Identification of the crop may be aided by the placement of a large gauge red rubber catheter down the esophagus. Severe crop burns may require such extensive surgical resection that only a small amount of crop tissue would be left to close [12]. In this situation, the prognosis for return to normal function would be poor [12]. Stents may be necessary for surgical closure. Another cause of trauma in birds is laceration or puncture of the caudal oropharynx, esophagus, or crop by rigid feeding cannulas [7].

Neoplasia

The occurrence of tumors in the esophagus or crop is considered rare [12]. Tumors of the esophagus and crop diagnosed in psittacine birds include squamous cell carcinoma and leiomyosarcoma [12]. Clinical signs of neoplasia include regurgitation, difficulty swallowing, and weight loss [12]. The presence of tumors may be diagnosed on physical examination, survey radiographs, contrast radiography, or endoscopy of the upper GI tract. Definitive diagnosis of neoplasia may be made with biopsy of lesions [12].

Papillomatosis

Papillomatosis, which has occurred in association with the esophagus and crop in Amazon parrots and macaws, will be discussed in detail under diseases of the cloaca [12].

Thyroid gland enlargement

In psittacine birds, a deficiency of iodine in the diet causes goiter, or hyperplasia of the thyroid gland [12]. Seed-based diets are deficient in iodine.Thyroid gland hyperplasia may cause enlargement of the thyroid glands that is not evident radiographically or on palpation [12]. Cockatiels and budgerigars are the most commonly reported species that develop goiter [12]. The proximity of the enlarged thyroid gland to the esophagus may interfere with the normal motility of the esophagus and crop [12]. This predisposes the bird to regurgitation, crop stasis, or crop distension due to mechanical impairment of motility [12]. Treatment of affected birds involves supplementation of seed-only diets with iodine or ideally conversion to a formulated diet. Related crop and esophageal disorders should be managed concurrently.

Heavy metal toxicosis

Poisoning with lead or zinc may lead to stasis of the esophagus and crop. Psittacine birds often become affected after ingestion of material composed of lead, zinc, or a combination of both metals. Toxicosis may be diagnosed with radiographs that show evidence of metal particles in the upper GI tract. Blood and tissue samples may be tested for heavy metal concentration. Treatment of heavy metal toxicosis is discussed in detail under diseases of the proventriculus and ventriculus.

Neuropathic gastric dilatation

This viral condition (also termed proventricular dilatation disease), causes myenteric ganglioneuritis of the GI tract, which may result in secondary stasis of the esophagus and crop [7,12]. Diagnosis and treatment will be discussed under diseases of the proventriculus and ventriculus.

Proventriculus and ventriculus

Neuropathic gastric dilatation

This disease is known by several synonyms, including proventricular dilatation disease, proventricular dilatation syndrome, and macaw wasting syndrome. Neuropathic gastric dilatation (NGD) causes infiltration of splanchnic nerves of the GI tract with lymphocytes and monocytes [7]. A variety of psittacine species, such as Amazon parrots, African gray parrots, cockatoos, conures, and cockatiels, have been affected by NGD [7]. Clinical signs of NGD include lethargy, anorexia, weight loss, neurological signs, regurgitation, or the passage of undigested seeds in the feces [7,12]. Peripheral neuritis in sciatic, brachial, and vagal nerves was also reported in a group of various psittacine birds with concurrent NGD [14]. Research on this disease suggests a viral etiology [7,12,20]. Other differentials for GI stasis, regurgitation, and a dilated proventriculus, such as heavy metal toxicosis, foreign bodies, neoplasia, or bacterial or fungal infection, should be ruled out as primary causes [12].

Presumptive diagnosis of NGD may be based upon history, clinical signs, and radiographs [12]. Blood work is typically unremarkable in these patients [12]. Some patients, however, may have nonspecific changes such as marked creatine phosphokinase elevation from weight loss or leucopenia indicating immunosuppression. Survey radiographs or contrast radiographs may show evidence of an abnormally dilated crop, proventriculus, ventriculus, or small intestine. However, in the early stages of the disease, the proventriculus may be a normal size radiographically [12]. A bird with more protracted disease may not need contrast media to determine the presence of a dilated proventriculus [7]. It should be noted that in neonates, the proventriculus is normally dilated [20].

A definitive diagnosis may be attempted with a biopsy of the GI tract such as the crop, proventriculus, or ventriculus [12]. On histopathology, NGD shows lymphocytic and plasmacytic infiltration of splanchnic nerves of the GI tract. A negative biopsy does not guarantee a bird is free of the disease if the biopsy was retrieved from a nondiagnostic area [7,12]. The risks of general anesthesia and potential surgical complications of hemorrhage and dehiscence with a gastric biopsy may preclude the ability to test for this disease [12]. A study of birds with NGD showed that only 67% of the crop biopsies exhibited the characteristic histopathologic changes [20].

Supportive care is the mainstay of treatment of NGD as birds cannot completely clear the infection. Affected birds may benefit from a warm incubator, gavage, parenteral fluids, systemic broad-spectrum antibiotic medications, antifungal medications, anti-inflammatory medications, and GI motility agents. The anti-inflammatory drug celecoxib (Celebrex; Pfizer; 10 mg/kg by mouth every 24 hours) has been used to prevent invasion of neurons by inflammatory cells [16]. Use of corticosteroid agents in avian patients is considered controversial due to the potential side effect of immunosuppression [12]. Prognosis for long-term survival is generally poor. The risk of transmission to naive birds is a strong possibility. Therefore, efforts should be made to keep these birds isolated from other birds when there is a high degree of suspicion of NGD. Current recommendations include the isolation, but not euthanasia, of exposed birds. Not all exposed birds have been shown to develop the disease [20].

Macrorhabdus ornithogaster *(formerly "megabacterium")*

Formerly referred to as megabacterium, *Macrorhabdus ornithogaster* is the newly proposed name of this previously undescribed anamorphic ascomycetous yeast, which represents a new genus [21]. This infectious organism may cause symptoms of lethargy, weight loss, emaciation, anorexia, regurgitation, vomiting, dark feces, and passing undigested seeds in the feces [7,22]. In budgerigars, these symptoms collectively have been described as a syndrome called "going light" [7,22]. *M ornithogaster* may cause disease in the proventriculus and the ventriculus [7,22]. Pathologic findings include proventriculitis, distention of the proventriculus, mucous buildup on the mucosal layer of the proventriculus, and thickening and hemorrhaging of the proventricular wall [7,22]. Despite repeated attempts, the pathogenicity of the organism is unclear due to an inability to find an avian model for infection and an inability to fulfill Koch's postulates [22,23].

Diagnosis of *M ornithogaster* in the liver bird may be made by identification of the organism in stained cytology of the feces or a proventricular wash [7,22]. *M ornithogaster* is a large (roughly 20–80 μm), rod-shaped, weakly Gram-positive, and periodic acid Schiff-positive organism [7,21,22]. Effective treatment in some bird species has been accomplished with oral amphotericin B for 30 days [22,24]. When given orally, amphotericin B is not absorbed by the GI tract, avoiding potential systemic side effects such as nephrotoxicity. Acidification of the proventriculus and supportive care with easily digestible food may also help resolve infection [22]. In one study, transmission of disease was prevented in budgerigars by removing eggs from the nest before hatching and hand-rearing the hatchlings [25].

Heavy metal toxicosis

Ingestion of heavy metal foreign bodies by psittacine birds may predispose them to development of zinc or lead toxicosis. Sources of lead poisoning include stained glass, curtain weights, Tiffany lamps, imported metal cages, or wall paint [18,26]. Zinc is a common ingredient of pennies minted since 1982, metallic household items like washers or nuts, and the powder found on newly galvanized cages [26,27]. Symptoms of heavy metal toxicosis include a dilated crop, crop stasis, regurgitation, weakness, anorexia, and weight loss. Seizures and other central nervous system signs may be seen in birds with lead poisoning. Erosions may result in gastritis, ulceration, or perforation of the ventriculus [12].

Diagnosis of heavy metal foreign bodies involves a thorough history and physical examination. Anemia and erythrocyte abnormalities, such as polychromatophilic red blood cells (RBC), hypochromic RBCs, and RBC nuclear abnormalities, may be detected on blood work [28]. Radiographs may show evidence of objects of heavy metal opacity in the ventriculus. However, lack of radiographically evident metal does not preclude the existence of heavy metal toxicosis. The blood should also be tested for evidence of elevated zinc and lead levels. Lead levels greater than 0.2 ppm and zinc levels above 2 ppm are diagnostic of toxicosis [27]. For accurate zinc level determination, it is critical that samples be placed in plastic containers or containers specially designed for determination of trace minerals [27,29]. However, these results should be considered along with the patient's clinical signs. Liver, kidney, and pancreatic tissue may also be tested for presence of elevated heavy metal levels, but these tests may be less than optimal to perform in the live patient.

Treatment of lead or zinc toxicosis will usually involve supportive care, including gavage, warm incubator, and parenteral fluids, especially in very critical patients. Anticonvulsant therapy may be indicated for patients with seizure activity [27,29,30]. Oral lubricating agents or bulk cathartics, such as mineral oil or peanut butter, may be helpful for removing smaller metal fragments from the ventriculus into the distal GI tract [27,30–32]. Radiography has been used to monitor the progress of metal pieces through the GI tract with less invasive techniques or to evaluate the success of more invasive methods when multiple metal pieces are involved [32].

Chelating agents are the mainstay of treatment in confirmed or suspected cases of heavy metal toxicosis. Zinc chelates faster than lead because unlike lead, it is not stored in bone [27,33]. Multiple treatments, or a break in treatment, may be needed because constant equilibration of heavy metals occurs during therapy [33]. Three commonly used chelators are D-penicillamine, calcium ethylenediaminetetraacetate (CaEDTA), and dimercaptosuccinic acid (DMSA) [34,35]. CaEDTA (35 mg/kg intramuscularly or subcutaneously every 12 hours for 5 days, off 3 to 4 days, then repeat as needed) has been the treatment of choice for heavy metal toxicosis in birds [10,33,34]. It must be given parenterally due to poor absorption from the GI tract [36]. Although it may be given intravenously, CaEDTA is typically given intramuscularly, and has been given subcutaneously at dilute concentrations [32,33]. CaEDTA may cause pain at the site of intramuscular injection [32]. Some veterinarians give CaEDTA for a maximum of 5 days with a 5- to 7-day rest period due to the potential for renal toxicity [33,36]. CaEDTA also does not reach therapeutic concentrations in the central nervous system [33].

DMSA (25–35 mg/kg by mouth every 12 h for 5 days/week for 3–5 weeks) and penicillamine (PA) (55 mg/kg by mouth every 12 h for 1–2 weeks) are oral chelators that may provide a safer alternative to CaEDTA [10,33]. DMSA and PA are reportedly less toxic and faster chelators than CaEDTA [26]. The major advantages of both drugs are reduced toxicity and potentially easier to treat oral formulations. Oral chelators, however, are contraindicated for use in vomiting birds [32]. DMSA and PA may also cause GI-related side effects such as regurgitation or vomiting [37]. The decision to use either an oral or parenteral chelator should be based upon the clinical signs of the bird.

When metal objects are large, they have the potential to perforate the ventriculus. These objects may require endoscopic or surgical retrieval [38]. Surgery of the ventriculus, however, has risks and potential complications. Another technique that involves flushing foreign objects out of the ventriculus and into the oral cavity for removal may be attempted [27]. Decontamination of heavy metal and other foreign bodies from the environment will go a long way toward preventing the occurrence or reoccurrence of heavy metal toxicosis.

Obstruction

Foreign substances ingested by psittacine birds are a relatively common cause of obstruction. Cage bedding, toys, string, grit, and other foreign materials like jewelry, appliance plugs, or wall baseboard are just some of the typical items reported to cause obstructions [17,39]. Other causes may not solely be the fault of the bird. For instance, a juvenile blue-and-gold macaw with an acute history of regurgitation, lethargy, and dehydration was discovered to have a gavage tube in its distal proventriculus [40]. Other symptoms of obstruction include anorexia, tenesmus, melena, and decreased defecations. Foreign materials may cause impaction or erosions of the proventriculus and ventriculus as well as secondary stasis of the GI tract [41,42]. The obstruction may not always be due to foreign material. One report diagnosed dysplastic koilin as the cause of proventricular obstruction in an eclectus parrot [43]. If indicated, treatment involves removal of the obstructing object with endoscopy or surgery.

Neoplasia

Gastric tumors are rare in psittacine birds [16]. The most common neoplasm reported is adenocarcinoma of the proventriculus or ventriculus [12,44]. The typical location for this tumor is along the isthmus, the area between the proventriculus and ventriculus [7,12]. Bile duct carcinoma and concurrent GI adenocarcinoma and papillomatosis have been reported in a peach-fronted conure [45]. Recent studies have provided evidence that herpes viruses—not papovavirus—may be associated with papillomatosis in some psittacine bird species [46,47].

Diagnosis of gastric tumors is based upon history, clinical signs, survey radiographs, or radiographs with contrast media. The history may suggest a change in the appetite of the bird. Clinical signs are usually nonspecific, including anorexia, regurgitation, weight loss, melena, and the passage of undigested seeds in the feces [7,12]. Blood work may show evidence of anemia, hypoproteinemia, and an elevated white cell count [7,12]. Contrast radiographs may show changes in the normal shape of the proventriculus or ventriculus or evidence of a filling defect. The tumor may be visualized with endoscopy of the proventriculus and ventriculus [7].

Treatment of patients suspected of having neoplasia involves supportive care. Surgical excision of the lesions or other tumors may be attempted but have the potential to be risky given the potential for hemorrhage and incision failure. The prognosis in most cases is considered to be poor. Gastric neoplasia complicated by hemorrhage may result in the eventual death of the patient if severe erosion of major blood vessels occurs [7,12].

Papillomatosis

Papillomatosis may occur in the upper GI tract [7]. Papillomatosis also occurs along the mucosal epithelial cell surfaces of the GI tract [16].

Small and large intestine

Ileus

Ileus occurs when there is decreased motility or complete stasis of the intestinal tract [7,12]. Causes of ileus include physical obstruction, impairment of intestinal nerves such as with neuropathic gastric dilatation, heavy metal toxicosis, peritonitis, or inflammation of the intestines [7,12]. Birds with ileus may exhibit signs of regurgitation, vomiting, decreased stool formation, and lethargy [7]. Intestinal obstruction may lead to loss of fluid from the circulation and subsequent fluid dilation of the intestinal lumen [7]. These avian patients will quickly become dehydrated and metabolically imbalanced [7,12]. Ischemic necrosis of the intestinal wall could lead to endotoxic shock from Gram-negative bacteria [7]. Blood work may show evidence of metabolic imbalance or increased hematocrit. Survey radiographs may show fluid- or gas-distended loops of bowel or a filling defect with contrast radiographs in the case of a foreign body obstruction [7]. Treatment involves supportive care in the case of NGD or surgical removal when a foreign body is suspected. A blue-and-gold macaw with a history of vomiting and producing small amounts of feces was diagnosed with a partially obstructive ileus that was successfully corrected with surgery [48].

Mycobacteriosis

Mycobacterium avium causes chronic wasting disease [12]. Infections with this bacteria have been reported in a number of psittacine species [29,49–54]. Transmission of this bacterial agent primarily occurs from contaminated feces via the fecal–oral route, but it can also occur through aerosolization [7,12]. This leads to bacterial colonization of the GI tract as well as the viscera [12]. Tubercles are formed in the intestinal wall that chronically shed acid-fast organisms [12]. Clinical signs include diarrhea, shifting leg lameness, and failure to thrive despite a good appetite [12]. The bacteria tend to be very hardy, and can persist in the environment for several months to several years [55].

Presumptive diagnosis of mycobacterial infection requires identification of acid-fast bacteria on appropriate stains of tissue or fecal samples [7]. A definitive diagnosis is obtained with biopsy, histopathology, and culture of affected tissue [55]. Culture has always been considered the "gold standard" for detection of *M avium*. A recent study in Japanese quail confirmed earlier studies that determined that both culture and polymerase chain reaction of tissue samples were more specific and sensitive for the detection of *M avium* compared with fecal sample evaluation [56]. Results of fecal sample evaluation may be most valuable with concurrent cultures [56].

Treatment of an *M avium* infection is generally not recommended due to the potential for shedding of the infectious agent into the environment and zoonotic potential [55]. Birds that come into contact with infected birds should be quarantined for at least 2 years and tested every 2 to 3 months for presence of antibodies to the disease [55]. After this time period, along with concurrent negative test results, birds may be considered free from disease [55]. Other mycobacterial species that affect birds include *M genevense* and *M tuberculosis*.

Enteritis

Intestinal infection with bacterial or fungal organisms may occur in psittacine birds as a primary infection or secondary to immunosuppression due to some other concurrent illness. Common causes of enteritis include *M ornithogaster*, *Clostridium* species, and *Campylobacter* species [12]. *Campylobacter* species are Gram-positive rods with variable forms that range from S- or spiral-shaped to comma-shaped [12]. *C jejuni* is considered the most pathogenic among the various species [12]. Diagnosis is based upon demonstration of light staining curved rods in feces, bile, or intestinal contents or culture [12]. Treatment is with systemic antimicrobial medication based upon culture and sensitivity results.

Clostridium species are another major cause of enteritis. In psittacine birds, they are considered an abnormal finding [57]. Clinical signs include vomiting, melena, lethargy, anorexia, diarrhea, regurgitation, and crop stasis [57,58]. Diagnosis is based upon stained cytology of the feces or isolation of the organism from the feces or the cloaca [12]. Treatment includes supportive care and antibiotic medications with a spectrum of activity against anaerobic bacteria. In this author's opinion, metronidazole (50 mg/kg by mouth every 12 h for 30 days) has been effective in the treatment of these infections [10]. Clindamycin and piperacillin have also been used for similar infections [57,58].

Cloaca

Cloacal prolapse

Prolapse of the cloaca may involve the oviduct, ureters, intestines, or coprodeum [7,12]. Cloacal prolapses may occur secondary to excessive straining during egg laying, excessive sexual behavior or, in the case of some cockatoos, as a result of idiopathic straining [12,16,59]. Cloacal prolapse occurred secondary to egg-related peritonitis in a blue-and-gold macaw [60]. Other causes include cloacitis, cloacaliths, or severe GI disease or obstruction [16]. The most prominent clinical sign is evidence of light to dark pink prolapsed cloacal tissue [7]. If prolapsed for an extended time, the tissue may become edematous, necrotic, or bloody from exposure or self traumatization [12]. When there is involvement from reproductive organs, such as the oviduct, the prolapsed tissue may have a cobblestone appearance.

Diagnosis of the cause of cloacal prolapse should be attempted, and will initially involve a thorough physical examination of the tissue [12,16]. Radiographs may identify any space-occupying lesions [12]. Treatment involves reduction of the prolapse under general anesthesia and the placement of lateral vent sutures [12,16]. Sutures should be placed so they do not interfere with the normal defecation or urination process [16]. Purse string-type suture placement is not recommended due to the potential for nerve damage of the vent sphincter. Recurrent cases of prolapsed cloaca may require ventplasty, cloacopexy, or salpingectomy in situations of chronic reproductive problems

[12,16,59]. However, without diagnosis of the underlying problem, these therapies may or may not resolve the cloacal prolapse.

Papillomatosis

Papillomatosis occurs commonly in the cloaca [12]. Studies have suggested that the causative agent may be a herpesvirus rather than a papovavirus, as was previously thought [46,61]. It has been reported in a variety of psittacine species [12]. Papillomatosis affects the mucosal layer of the cloaca where lesions may be focal or extend the circumference of the cloaca [12]. Occasionally, lesions may be too deep to identify [12]. More advanced lesions are characterized by raspberry-like tissue that is either red or pink in color [7]. Symptoms of papillomatosis include cloacitis, melena, foul-smelling feces, tenesmus, flatulence, a pasty vent, and bleeding lesions [7,16].

A presumptive diagnosis of papillomatosis may be based upon the appearance of raspberry-shaped lesions [12]. These lesions, however, may be sometimes be confused with a prolapsed cloaca [7,12]. Application of acetic acid will turn these lesions white [7,12]. A biopsy of the lesion will provide a definitive diagnosis [7,12]. Papillomatosis is challenging to treat due to the likelihood of spontaneous reoccurrence [7,12]. A variety of techniques, from radiosurgery and cryosurgery to chemical cauterization, have been attempted with varying degrees of success [7,12]. Some clinicians will not treat papillomatosis unless clinical signs like discomfort and bleeding are severe enough to warrant treatment [12].

The anatomy and physiology of the avian GI tract offers insight into the normal function of this organ system. The diagnosis and treatment of psittacine GI disorders requires an understanding of this anatomy and physiology as well as a thorough evaluation of the history and clinical signs of the avian patient. Although some diseases such as lead toxicosis may be treated, others such as neoplasia and neuropathic gastric dilatation may not, and may carry a poor prognosis for normal return to function. The avian practitioner can use a combination of the clues provided by the patient's clinical signs and diagnostic test results to adequately determine the prognosis in each case.

References

[1] Denbow DM. Gastrointestinal anatomy and physiology. In: Whittow GC, editor. Sturkie's avian physiology. 5th edition. Boston: Academic Press; 2000. p. 299–326.
[2] King AS, McLelland J. Birds their structure and function. Philadelphia: Bailliere Tindall; 1984.
[3] McMillan MC. Imaging techniques. In: Ritchie BW, Harrison GJ, Harrison LR, editors. Avian medicine: principles and application. Lake Worth (FL): Wingers Publishing Inc.; 1994. p. 246–326.
[4] Goldstein DL, Skadhauge E. Renal and extrarenal regulation of body fluid composition. In: Whittow GC, editor. Sturkie's avian physiology. 5th edition. New York: Academic Press; 2000. p. 265–98.

[5] Gerlach H. Viruses. In: Ritchie BW, Harrison GJ, Harrison LR, editors. Avian medicine: principles and application. Lake Worth (FL): Wingers Publishing Inc.; 1994. p. 862–948.

[6] Ritchie BW. Avian viruses: function and control. Lake Worth (FL): Wingers Publishing Inc.; 1995.

[7] Lumeij JT. Gastroenterology. In: Ritchie BW, Harrison GJ, Harrison LR, editors. Avian medicine: principles and application. Lake Worth (FL): Wingers Publishing Inc.; 1994. p. 482–521.

[8] Zwijnenberg RJ, Zwart P. Squamous metaplasia in the salivary glands of canaries (a case report). Vet Q 1994;16(1):60–1.

[9] Harrison GJ, Ritchie BW. Making distinctions in the physical examination. In: Ritchie BW, Harrison GJ, Harrison LR, editors. Avian medicine: principles and application. Lake Worth (FL): Wingers Publishing Inc.; 1994. p. 144–75.

[10] Carpenter JW, Mashima TY, Rupiper DJ. Exotic animal formulary. 2nd edition. Philadelphia: WB Saunders; 2001.

[11] Koutsos EA, Tell LA, Woods LW, et al. Adult cockatiels (Nymphicus hollandicus) at maintenance are more sensitive to diets containing excess vitamin A than to vitamin A-deficient diets. J Nutr 2003;133(6):1898–902.

[12] Hoefer HL. Diseases of the gastrointestinal tract. In: Altman RB, Clubb SL, Dorrestein GM, Quesenberry KE, editors. Avian medicine and surgery. Philadelphia: WB Saunders; 1997. p. 419–53.

[13] Anderson NL. Recurrent deep foreign body granuloma in the tongue of an African grey parrot (Psittacus erithacus timneh). J Avian Med Surg 1997;11(2):105–9.

[14] Berhane Y, Smith DA, Newman S, et al. Peripheral neuritis in psittacine birds with proventricular dilatation disease. Avian Pathol 2001;30(5):563–70.

[15] Harris DJ, Roston MA, Marx KL. Medical management of crop stasis. Paper presented at the proceedings of the 20th annual conference on avian medicine and surgery Mid Atlantic States Association of Avian Veterinarians, Baltimore, MD, USA, 25–27 April, 1999. p. 81–84.

[16] Girling S. Diseases of the digestive tract of psittacine birds. In Pract 2004;26(3):146–53.

[17] Oglesbee B, Steinohrt L. Gastrointestinal string foreign bodies in a juvenile umbrella cockatoo. Compend Contin Educ Pract Vet 2001;23(11):946–50, 974.

[18] Archambault AL, Timm KI. Treatment of acute lead ingestion in a juvenile macaw. J Am Vet Med Assoc 1994;205(6):852–4.

[19] Harrison GJ. Indications for an ingluviotomy. Exotic DVM 2000;2:6.

[20] Gregory CR. Proventricular dilatation disease. In: Ritchie BW, editor. Avian viruses: function and control. Lake Worth (FL): Wingers Publishing Inc.; 1995. p. 439–48.

[21] Tomaszewski EK, Logan KS, Snowden KF, et al. Phylogenetic analysis identifies the "megabacterium" of birds as a novel anamorphic ascomycetous yeast, Macrorhabdus ornithogaster gen. nov., sp. nov. Int J Syst Evol Microbiol 2003;53(Pt 4):1201–5.

[22] Dorrestein GM. Bacteriology. In: Altman RB, Clubb SL, Dorrestein GM, Quesenberry KE, editors. Avian medicine and surgery. Philadelphia: WB Saunders; 1997. p. 255–80.

[23] Phalen DN, Moore RP. Experimental infection of white-leghorn cockerels with Macrorhabdos ornithogaster (Megabacterium). Avian Dis 2003;47(2):254–60.

[24] Gestier AW, Marx KL, Roston MA. Treatment of megabacteria in Budgerigars by in-water medication with soluble Amphotericin B. Paper presented at the proceedings of the 23rd annual conference on avian medicine and surgery. Mid Atlantic States Association of Avian Veterinarians, Fredericksburg, VA, USA, 28–30 April 2002. p. 173–5.

[25] Moore RP, Snowden KF, Phalen DN. A method of preventing transmission of so-called "megabacteria" in budgerigars (Melopsittacus undulatus). J Avian Med Surg 2001;15(4): 283–7.

[26] Holz P, Phelan J, Slocombe R, et al. Suspected zinc toxicosis as a cause of sudden death in orange-bellied parrots (Neophema chrysogaster). J Avian Med Surg 2000;14(1):37–41.

[27] Bauck L, LaBonde J. Toxic diseases. In: Altman RB, Clubb SL, Dorrestein GM, Quesenberry KE, editors. Avian medicine and surgery. Philadelphia: WB Saunders; 1997. p. 604–13.

[28] Christopher MM, Shooshtari MP, Levengood JM. Assessment of erythrocyte morphologic abnormalities in mallards with experimentally induced zinc toxicosis. Am J Vet Res 2004; 65(4):440–6.

[29] Ritzman TK, Hawley SB. What is your diagnosis? Mycobacterial infection and zinc toxicosis in a pionus parrot (Pionus senilis). J Avian Med Surg 1997;11(3):211–4.

[30] Riggs SM, Puschner B, Tell LA. Management of an ingested lead foreign body in an Amazon parrot. Vet Hum Toxicol 2002;44(6):345–8.

[31] Droual R, Meteyer CU, Galey FD. Zinc toxicosis due to ingestion of a penny in a gray-headed chachalaca (Ortalis cinereiceps). Avian Dis 1991;35(4):1007–11.

[32] Jenkins JR. Avian critical care and medicine. In: Altman RB, Clubb SL, Dorrestein GM, Quesenberry K, editors. Avian medicine and surgery. Philadelphia: WB Saunders; 1997. p. 839–64.

[33] Tully TN Jr, Hoefer H, Vansant F, et al. Heavy metal toxicosis. J Avian Med Surg 1997; 11(2):115–8.

[34] Denver MC, Tell LA, Galey FD, et al. Comparison of two heavy metal chelators for treatment of lead toxicosis in cockatiels. Am J Vet Res 2000;61(8):935–40.

[35] Hoogesteijn AL, Raphael BL, Calle P, et al. Oral treatment of avian lead intoxication with meso-2,3-dimercaptosuccinic acid. J Zoo Wildl Med 2003;34(1):82–7.

[36] Ryan T. Zinc toxicity in a cockatiel. Paper presented at the Mid-Atlantic States Association of Avian Veterinarians, Clinton, MD, 1997.

[37] Speer BL. Observations of basic diagnostic profile patterns seen in some common disorders of backyard poultry species. Vet Clin North Am Exotic Anim Pract 1999;2:701–8.

[38] Miller MA, Weber MA. Clinical challenge. Metallic foreign body in the region of the proventriculus. J Zoo Wildl Med 2000;31(4):578–80.

[39] Adamcak A, Hess LR, Quesenberry KE. Intestinal string foreign body in an adult umbrella cockatoo (Cacatua alba). J Avian Med Surg 2000;14(4):257–63.

[40] Rich G. What is your diagnosis? Ingested foreign body in a macaw (Ara aracauna). J Avian Med Surg 1995;9(2):145–6.

[41] Morris JM, Lemarchand T, Oliver J, et al. What is your diagnosis? Foreign body in a sulfur crested cockatoo, Cacatua galerita. J Avian Med Surg 1995;9(3):199–201.

[42] Speer BL. Chronic partial proventricular obstruction caused by multiple gastrointestinal foreign bodies in a juvenile umbrella cockatoo (Cacatua alba). J Avian Med Surg 1998;12(4): 271–5.

[43] Voe RD, Degernes L, Karli K, et al. Dysplastic koilin causing proventricular obstruction in an eclectus parrot (Eclectus roratus). J Avian Med Surg 2003;17(1):27–32.

[44] Yonemaru K, Sakai H, Asaoka Y, et al. Proventricular adenocarcinoma in a Humboldt penguin (Spheniscus humboldti) and a great horned owl (Bubo virginianus); identification of origin by mucin histochemistry. Avian Pathol 2004;33(1):77–81.

[45] Gibbons PM, Busch MD, Tell LA, et al. Internal papillomatosis with intrahepatic cholangiocarcinoma and gastrointestinal adenocarcinoma in a peach-fronted conure (Aratinga aurea). Avian Dis 2002;46(4):1062–9.

[46] Styles DK, Tomaszewski EK, Jaeger LA, et al. Psittacid herpesviruses associated with mucosal papillomas in neotropical parrots. Virology 2004;325(1):24–35.

[47] Johne R, Konrath A, Krautwald-Junghanns ME, et al. Herpesviral, but no papovaviral sequences, are detected in cloacal papillomas of parrots. Arch Virol 2002;147(10):1869–80.

[48] Horst HVD, Kirpestein J, Wolvekamp P, et al. Surgical correction of ileus in a blue-and-gold macaw (Ara ararauna). Avian Dis 1996;40(2):484–7.

[49] Hoop RK. Mycobacterium tuberculosis infection in a canary (Serinus canana L.) and a blue-fronted Amazon parrot (Amazona amazona aestiva). Avian Dis 2002;46(2):502–4.

[50] Worell AB. Cutaneous mycobacteriosis in a Moluccan cockatoo. Exotic Pet Pract 2000; 5(1):7.

[51] Rich G. Avian mycobacterial infection. Exotic Pet Pract 2000;5(6):47.

[52] Washko RM, Hoefer H, Kiehn TE, et al. Mycobacterium tuberculosis infection in a green-winged macaw (Ara chloroptera): report with public health implications. J Clin Microbiol 1998;36(4):1101–2.

[53] Rich G, Evans D, Bone T, et al. What is your diagnosis? Mycobacteriosis in an Amazon parrot (Amazona amazonica). J Avian Med Surg 1997;11(3):206–10.

[54] Tully TN, Morris JM, Pechman RD, et al. What is your diagnosis? Tuberculosis in an Amazon parrot. J Avian Med Surg 1995;9(1):57–8.

[55] Gerlach H. Bacteria. In: Ritchie BW, Harrison GJ, Harrison LR, editors. Avian medicine: principles and application. Lake Worth (FK): Wingers Publishing Inc.; 1994. p. 949–83.

[56] Tell LA, Foley J, Needham ML, et al. Diagnosis of avian mycobacteriosis: comparison of culture, acid-fast stains, and polymerase chain reaction for the identification of Mycobacterium avium in experimentally inoculated Japanese quail (Coturnix coturnix japonica). Avian Dis 2003;47(2):444–52.

[57] Ferrell ST, Tell L. Clostridium tertium infection in a rainbow lorikeet (Trichoglossus haematodus haematodus) with enteritis. J Avian Med Surg 2001;15(3):204–8.

[58] Wilson GH, Fontenot DK, Greenacre CB, et al. Enteric clostridial colonization in psittacine birds. Compend Contin Educ Pract Vet 2002;24(7):550–4.

[59] Worell AB. Cloacal prolapse in an umbrella cockatoo. Exotic Pet Pract 1998;3(6):47.

[60] Wilson H, Graham J. Management of egg-related peritonitis in a blue and gold macaw (Ara ararauna). Compend Contin Educ Pract Vet 2003;25(1):42–7.

[61] Johne R, Konrath A, Krautwald Junghanns ME, et al. Herpesviral, but no papovaviral sequences, are detected in cloacal papillomas of parrots. Arch Virol 2002;147(10):1869–80.

ELSEVIER
SAUNDERS

Vet Clin Exot Anim 8 (2005) 351–375

VETERINARY
CLINICS
Exotic Animal Practice

Rabbit Gastroenterology

Brigitte Reusch, BVetMed (Hons), MRCVS

Small Animal Hospital, University of Bristol, Division of Companion Animals,
Department of Clinical Veterinary Science, Langford, Bristol BS40 4DU, UK

Gastroenterology of the rabbit has been well studied, and includes the gastrointestinal tract and its disorders. Pet rabbits are often presented with anorexia, weight loss, changes in defecation, and depression. Diet-related disease and stress-related disease, resulting in immunosuppression and decreased gastrointestinal motility, predominate, and can play a large role in preventative medicine.

This article presents an overview of common gastrointestinal disorders and emergency concerns, which should be considered when the small animal practitioner is presented with a rabbit patient.

Disorders of the oral cavity and esophagus

Dental disease

Etiology

A comprehensive review of the etiology and treatment of dental disease in the rabbit is beyond the scope of this article. There are several causes of malocclusion, which is the most common dental abnormality seen in pet rabbits. Congenital deformity, trauma, dietary problems, and neoplasia (eg, mandibular osteosarcoma) are also seen [1]. Mandibular and maxillary abscesses associated with dental infections are common. Periodontal disease and pulpitis are often involved, especially in cases of iatrogenic longitudinal fractures caused by teeth clipping.

Clinical features

Congenital malocclusion first presents at 8 to 10 weeks of age, although may only be noticed at 12 to 18 months of age [2]. Osteosarcoma, rarely reported in the rabbit, seen mainly over 6 years of age, although has been

E-mail address: B.Reusch@bristol.ac.uk

reported in an 18-month-old [1,3]. Anorexia, dysphagia, bruxism due to pain, ptyalism with secondary moist dermatitis, halitosis, epiphora, weight loss, reduction in size or amount of fecal pellets, reduction in ingestion of caecotrophs, abscesses, or facial swelling development may all be signs of dental disease. Pyrexia is not usually seen with abscesses in rabbits.

Diagnosis

Dental disease is usually first suspected on history and clinical findings. Oral examination may reveal some dental and soft tissue changes, but radiography is recommended to evaluate disease of the roots and surrounding alveolar bone. Radiolucent periapical regions due to bone lysis and abscess formation and periosteal bone reaction may be identified on radiography. Marked increases in serum alkaline phosphatase, approximately two times the normal value, has been documented in cases of skeletal osteosarcoma [3].

Treatment and prognosis

Depending on the primary cause of dental disease, corrective burring or extraction of affected teeth, supportive care, and diet change to higher fiber diet may be indicated. Complete surgical excision is the recommended treatment of abscesses in the rabbit; however, this is not usually possible in periapical abscesses. Debridement and extraction of associated teeth is recommended. Systemic and local antibiosis should be based on culture and sensitivity. Antibiotic-impregnated polymethylmethacrylate beads can be placed in the debrided abscess, and depending on the choice of antibiotic, can maintain antibiotic levels above the minimum inhibitory concentration for a minimum of 7 days, but at least 30 days for gentamicin- and amikacin-impregnated beads [4,5].

Mandibulectomy only, in dogs with mandibular osteosarcoma, has a 1-year survival rate of 71% [6]. Metastasis of the thoracic and abdominal viscera has been reported in rabbits [1,7–9]. As the biologic behavior of this neoplasm in rabbits is not fully known, surgical excision and chemotherapy would be the most aggressive treatment. Euthanasia is indicated with metastatic disease cases.

Prognosis of dental disease is dependent on the primary cause and extent of secondary changes. If there is radiographic evidence of osteomyelitis, the prognosis is guarded to poor.

Oral papillomatosis

Etiology

Oral papillomaviruses cause hyperproliferative lesions of the oral mucosa in rabbits. Natural infection in the domestic rabbit has been sporadically reported, often as an incidental finding at necropsy. Lesions are principally found in rabbits less than 2 years of age. Frequency of oral papillomas approached one third, regardless of age and sex in one study of New Zealand white rabbits examined from two local sources [10]. This was higher than the frequency in previous reports of 5% in New Zealand white rabbits [11] and 16.6% in Giant Checkers, California, New Zealand white and red, Angora, Dutch belted blue, and brown and Sable [12].

Clinical features

Papillomas occur mainly on the ventral tongue surface, occasionally tongue tip, and grossly appear as white, 1 to 3-mm plaques [10]. In one report maximum growth was at 3 to 4 weeks postinfection, with natural regression by 6 to 8 weeks [13].

Diagnosis

Biopsy and histopathology are required for a definitive diagnosis.

Treatment and prognosis

Specific treatment has not been described; however, supportive treatment for discomfort or secondary infection may be indicated. Spontaneous resolution and subsequent immunity offers a good prognosis. A feasible and effective multiple-antigen peptide vaccine for the prevention of papillomavirus infection has been developed, but is not commercially available [13].

Sialoadenitis and salivary gland necrosis

Etiology

The etiology is unknown, but the condition has been found in a 16-month-old crossbreed rabbit, at postmortem examination. (J.M. Bradshaw, personal communication).

Clinical features

Painless enlargement of one or more salivary glands may be seen with this condition. Dysphagia and discomfort may be present if there is extensive inflammation.

Diagnosis

Fine-needle aspirate and cytology or biopsy and histopathology can confirm the mass is salivary tissue and whether inflammation or necrosis is present.

Treatment and prognosis

Analgesia and anti-inflammatory therapy are indicated if pain or dysphagia is present, although surgical resection may be ultimately required. Further investigation in rabbits is indicated; however, prognosis in cats and dogs is usually excellent [13].

Esophagitis

Etiology

Principally, esophagitis is caused by gastroesophageal reflux, persistent vomiting, ingestion of caustic agents, or esophageal foreign objects in the cat and dog [14]. The rabbit presumably does not, or cannot, vomit due to a well-developed cardiac sphincter [15,16]. However, evidence of regurgitation, with secondary aspiration of food into the trachea and lungs, was found on several postmortem examinations [17].

Clinical features

The rabbit is used as a model for human esophagitis, where in one study esophagitis was induced by acidified pepsin perfusion. Lesions observed in acute and chronic low-grade esophagitis in the rabbit model included mucosal/submucosal bleeding, erosions, ulcers, and hyperemia. Evidence of esophageal mucosal adaptation was found; the suggested mechanism for this was cell proliferation [18]. A smaller subepithelial mast cells population and decreased inflammatory mediator release was also found to attribute to rabbit esophageal mucosa resistance [19]. Clinically, 523 ± 132 g weight loss was seen in rabbits with esophagitis compared with 78 ± 26 g in those with no damage [18]. Anorexia and ptyalism may be seen if swallowing is painful. Where a caustic agent has been ingested, the mouth and tongue are hyperemic and often ulcerated, with marked acute anorexia.

Diagnosis

Plain and contrast radiographs may reveal esophageal foreign bodies. In most cases endoscopy with or with out biopsy is needed for definitive diagnosis of esophagitis, as contrast esophagrams are unreliable.

Treatment and prognosis

Sucralfate (Antepsin) (25 mg/kg orally every 8–12 hours) either a crushed tablet slurry or viscous gel has been shown to bind to pepsin substrates in tissues, resulting in very effective prevention of experimentally induced peptic esophagitis in rabbits. In cases where gastric reflux is suspected, an antacid should be administered. H_2 receptor antagonists will reduce gastric acid, and have also been shown to have concentration-dependent prokinetic effects on the rabbit stomach fundus and sigmoid colon; the order of potency was ranitidine $>$ famotidine $>$ cimetidine [20]. Analgesia is indicated; however, caution with nonsteroidal anti-inflammatory drugs (NSAIDS) would seem sensible. The author's preference is buprenorphine (Vetergesic) (0.01–0.05 mg/kg, subcutaneously, every 6–8 hours) because of its long duration of action. Gastrotomy feeding tubes may be required in severe cases to allow optimum mucosal healing while preventing ileus and hepatic lipidosis. Antibiotics effective against anaerobes (eg, metronidazole) may be indicated. Further investigation into the incidence, etiology, and prognosis of spontaneous esophagitis is required. Prognosis will be dependent on the severity of esophagitis and whether the primary cause can be addressed. Early and aggressive therapy may help prevent stricture formation. Foreign bodies with secondary perforations have a grave prognosis.

Disorders of the stomach

Gastric ulceration

Etiology and clinical features
Gastric ulceration was observed in 7.3% (n = 1000) of rabbits, at postmortem examination [21]. Fundic ulceration was a relatively common finding (53 of 73 cases), and these rabbits were also found to have other clinically significant disease, including anorexia, enteritis, typhilitis, intussusception, and bronchopneumonia [21]. Prevalence increased with age (15% were over 2 years of age), and was also seen more commonly in females. A suggested etiology was stress-induced ulceration, as a consequence of stress of disease [21]. Similar lesions were reproduced with intraperitoneal injection of adrenaline, in rabbits [22]. Another mechanism for fundic ulceration is hypovolemic shock, where lesions can develop with in 3 hours [23]. Fundic ulcers occurred as small, multiple, shallow erosions of the gastric mucosa, and none were perforated [21].

Pyloric ulcers mainly occurred as single lesions, up to 1 cm in diameter. Perforation and peritonitis was associated in 70% of the pyloric ulceration cases, and this was the only lesion of clinical significance found at postmortem examination. Only one case was associated with gastric impaction; the others mainly died during parturition or in the immediate postparturient period. Peak incidence was in 6- to 9-month-old rabbits (60% of total cases). The abdominal contractions during parturition may have precipitated the gastric perforations in these cases [21]. Of the histologic sections examined, no bacterial infection or presence of fungi were found in both fundic and pyloric ulcerations.

Anorexia can be the principle sign, bruxism, and affected rabbits may be reluctant to move, indicating severe pain. Melena is seldom seen in the rabbit. In some cases clinical signs due to anemia and hypoproteinemia may be seen (pale mucous membranes, dyspnoea, weakness, collapse, and shock). Some ulcers may perforate and then seal rapidly by adhesions, forming abscesses with in the gastric wall. Aspirin-induced acute gastric ulceration occurred in a rabbit used in a pharmacologic study [24].

Diagnosis
Signs of acute abdomen and sepsis may be seen in rabbits with perforation and peritonitis, and there may be evidence of peritonitis on plain radiography. Ultrasonography can be useful in detecting gastric wall thickening associated with infiltrative disease (eg, lymphoma [25]).

Endoscopy is the most sensitive and specific tool for diagnosing gastric ulceration, although in most cases the rabbit is unlikely to be stable enough for general anesthesia at the time of presentation.

Treatment and prognosis

Therapy depends on the severity of the ulceration and whether the underlying cause is detected. Rabbits with perforation and peritonitis have a very grave prognosis. Symptomatic or prophylactic treatment could be considered in higher risk cases such as females in late gestation, rabbits with anorexia, enteritis, or chronic disease. This would include decreasing acid production, protecting ulcerated mucosa, fluid therapy, analgesia, antibiosis, and supportive nutrition. Omeprazole has been shown to completely inhibit basal acid secretion and elevate postprandial intragastric from to pH above 5.0 in rabbits. Ranitidine partially inhibited basal acid secretion (73%), and partially decreased pepsin secretion (37%) [26]. Cimetidine, however, was found to be ineffective in protecting against stress-related gastric lesions in a rabbit model [22]. Sucralfate may be effective in treating gastric ulceration.

Gastric stasis and gastrointestinal ileus

Etiology

Gastric stasis is primarily an acquired disorder of decreased motility. Generalized ileus is a common continuation of this condition, and may arise from mechanical obstruction or from defective propulsion. Mechanical obstruction (eg, dehydrated impacted ingesta secondary to chronic dehydration, foreign bodies, and infiltrative lesions) cause delayed gastric empting. Abnormalities in myenteric neuronal or gastric smooth muscle function or contractility result in defective propulsion. Primary factors associated with these functional disorders include anorexia, high-carbohydrate/low-fiber diet, postsurgical adhesions, lack of exercise, toxin ingestion (lead). Secondary factors include pain and environmental stressors such as proximity of predators or a dominant rabbit, change in group hierarchy, loss of a companion, change in housing, routine, or diet, transport, extremes of temperatures, or humidity [27]. Anorexia and chronic dehydration are both causal factors and consequences of gastric stasis and ileus. Systemic dehydration leads to gut content dehydration and impaction of normal stomach contents, which includes loose hair lattices or trichobezoars. One study found the prevalence of trichobezoars, weighing 1 to 24 g, to be 23.1% (n = 208) [16].

Clinical features

Gradual decrease in appetite leading to anorexia (days–weeks), decreased size and amount of fecal pellets, gradual progression from bright and alert to depression, dehydration, and death.

Diagnosis

The history and clinical findings of a firm, dough-like stomach on palpation, allow a presumptive diagnosis of gastric stasis and ileus, and are suggestive of nonobstructive disease. Although advanced cases do not permit differentiation between obstructive and nonobstructive stasis and ileus. Plain radiography in early cases reveals a mass of hair and food, appearing similar to normal ingesta. As the impaction in the stomach and occasionally cecum develops, a gas halo is often seen around the compacted material (Fig. 1). Large amounts of gas are seen through out the gastrointestinal tract (GIT) as a result of ileus (Figs. 1 and 2). A definitive diagnosis can only be made on exploratory laparotomy; however, this is a high-risk procedure in these already metabolically unstable rabbits.

Treatment and prognosis

Aggressive medical management is required to prevent further deterioration and death. Nearly 10% of fundic ulcers were found to be associated with anorexia or cecal impaction in a survey of gastric ulceration in the rabbit [21]. Hepatic lipidosis is a common complication and cause of death in rabbits, with prolonged gastric stasis and ileus. Rehydration, of both the patient and stomach contents, with both oral and intravenous fluids, may be required depending on the severity of the case; 100 mL/kg/d is the maintenance volume in the rabbit.

Analgesics, such as buprenorphine (0.01–0.05 mg/kg, subcutaneously, every 6–8 hours) or butorphanol (Torbujesic) (0.1–0.5 mg/kg subcutaneously or intravenously, every 2–4 hours), in the first instance, and then once rehydrated, NSAIDS, for example, meloxicam (Metacam) (0.1–0.6 mg/kg subcutaneously or orally, every 24 hours) [28] or carprofen (Rimadyl)

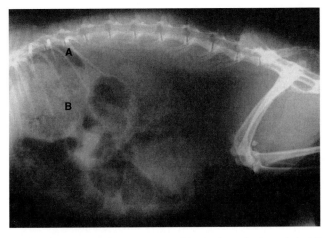

Fig. 1. Lateral abdominal radiograph of a rabbit with gastric stasis. A gas halo (*A*) can be seen around the compacted ingesta within the stomach (*B*).

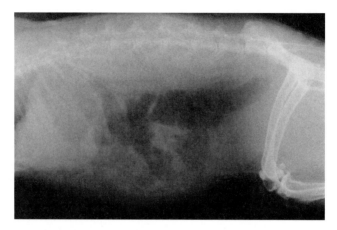

Fig. 2. Lateral abdominal radiograph of a rabbit with generalized ileus, large amounts of gas can be seen within the small and large intestines. The stomach reveals a mass of ingesta, similar in appearance to the normal rabbit stomach.

(2–4 mg/kg subcutaneously, intravenously or orally, every 24 hours) are also appropriate.

Prokinetics are required to stimulate GIT motility. Cisapride (Prepulsid) (0.5 mg/kg orally every 8–12 hours) a potent prokinetic, acts on 5-hydroxytryptamine (5-HT or serotonin) receptors and facilitates and restores motility throughout the length of the GIT. Dosing intervals for cisapride should be every 8 hours, as the plasma half-life was found to be 4 to 10 hours in the rabbit [29]. Cisapride was withdrawn in 2000, from several Western European countries, the United States, and Canada, because it was shown to be associated with a rare, but potentially fatal ventricular arrhythmia (Torsade de pointes) in humans, due to drug-induced delayed repolarization and prolongation of the QT wave interval. Similar characteristics have been characterized in rabbit hearts and canine cardiac Purkinje fiber, but in vivo effects have not yet been reported in dogs, cats, or rabbits [30–32].

Metoclopramide (Emequel) (0.5 mg/kg orally or subcutaneously every 8–24 hours), is a dopamine antagonist having both central (antiemetic and depressant) and peripheral (prokinetic) effects. The prokinetic effects of metoclopramide are not as potent as cisapride and are limited to the proximal GIT. Having prokinetic effects equal to cisapride [33], and antacid actions makes ranitidine (Zantac) (2–5 mg/kg orally every 12–24 hours) a very useful drug, in the author's opinion, in the treatment of gastric stasis and ileus.

Experimental prokinetics, which have been shown to effectively stimulate the rabbit GIT include motilin analogs (KW-5139) [34], a structurally related compound to metoclopramide (6-chloro-2,3-dihydro-4(1H)-quinazolinone derivatives), this compares favorably with cisapride [35], and a prokinetic macrolide derived from erythromycin (EM574) [36].

Dimethicone (Infacol; 20–40 mg/kg orally every 6 hours) may be useful if a large amount of gas is present. Exercise will also stimulate GIT motility and should be encouraged.

Nutritional support to reverse energy balance and stimulate motility can be achieved by syringe feeding commercially available high fiber recovery diets, for example, Critical Care for Herbivores (Oxbow Petlife International Ltd., Bury St. Edmunds, Suffolk, UK), ground up rabbit pellets or pureed vegetables and grass, four to five times a day. A wide variety of fresh vegetation should be offered daily, to encourage the rabbit to eat. Nasogastric tubes are easily placed in a conscious calm or weak rabbit, in a similar manner to that used in a cat. Radiography is always recommended to ensure the tube is in the correct position (Fig. 3). Some rabbits will tolerate the tube without an Elizabethan collar, which will enable eating, caecotrophy, and is less stressful (Fig. 4). Blended and strained food can then be fed, flushing with 5 mL of water before and after feeding will keep the tube patent. Nasogastric tubes can be left in place for several days. Antibiotic therapy such as enrofloxacin (Baytril; 10–30 mg/kg orally subcutaneously, every 24 hours) is advisable to help prevent rhinitis, which may develop if nasal tissue was traumatized.

A technique for placing pharyngostomy tubes in the laboratory rabbit has been described. This was modeled on the technique used in cats and dogs, with the adaptation of a subcutaneous tunnel from the pharyngotomy incision to the posterior base of the ear, there by eliminating the need for an Elizabethan collar. Tubes remained in place for 6 to 12 months, and only 2 of 40 rabbits developed abscesses along the subcutaneous tunnel. No disturbance in eating, drinking, or weight gain was noted over the 12-month period; no sepsis occurred at the exit point, by the ear, after removal of the catheter [37].

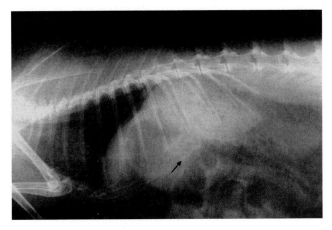

Fig. 3. Lateral thoracoabdominal radiograph of a rabbit, confirming correct placement of a nasogastric tube (*arrow*).

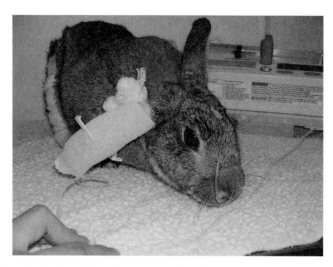

Fig. 4. Photograph of a rabbit with a nasogastric tube secured to the head with glue. This rabbit did not require an Elizabethan collar.

Endoscopic placement of percutaneous gastrotomy tubes was performed in five laboratory rabbits [38]. Elizabethan collars and jackets were poorly tolerated by most of the rabbits and superficial necrosis or purulent exudate around the percutaneous gastrotomy tube incisions occurred from day 4 of the study in four of the rabbits [38]. This technique does not appear to be as useful in rabbits as it is in cats and dogs.

Gastric obstruction

Etiology

Ingested objects such as matted hair, carpet, plastic, or rubber, can pass down the esophagus and become a gastric or intestinal foreign body. The pylorus is a common site of obstruction, and material or objects lodged in this area can cause gastric outflow obstruction.

Clinical features

The rabbit patient with gastric obstruction may be asymptomatic or have anorexia initially until an acute abdomen rapidly develops (24–48 hours). A sudden lack of defaecation, enlarged tympanic abdomen, or signs of abdominal pain can develop, followed by hypovolemia and shock characterized by tachycardia, tachypnea, pale, tacky mucous membranes, slow capillary refill time, bounding to weak peripheral pulses, hypothermia, or collapse. Hepatic lipidosis is a common accompanying lesion in gastric obstruction [39]. Death often occurs with in 24–48 hours. Liver lobe torsion, of the left lobe or caudate lobe has been reported in the rabbit, and may present with an acute abdomen, or sudden death [40].

Diagnosis

Clinical signs are usually indicative, but obstructions can rarely be detected on abdominal palpation alone, and there is a high risk of trauma to the distended stomach and friable liver (secondary to hepatic lipidosis). Plain radiography often is often nondiagnostic, although fluid and gas cranial to the obstruction and gas bubbles with in the stomach may be seen. Serial plain radiography can reveal signs of obstruction. Contrast studies can be difficult to interpret due to the normal presence of ingesta always in the stomach and cecum, gas in the intestines, cecum, and colon, and recirculation of barium if coprophagia occurs. In most cases, exploratory laparotomy is required for diagnosis.

Treatment and prognosis

Aggressive treatment is essential in this life-threatening condition. Stabilization of the rabbit before gastrotomy is essential to optimize a successful outcome. Analgesia, the author's preference, is for buprenorphine or pethidine (Pethidine; 5–10 mg/kg intramuscularly or subcutaneously), shock doses of intravenous or intraosseous crystalloid solution, and systemic broad-spectrum antibiotics should be administered. Prokinetics are contraindicated with an obstructive condition before surgery, but are useful postoperatively to stimulate gastrointestinal motility. Gastric decompression via nasogastric or orogastric tube should always be attempted. Where possible serum electrolyte concentrations and acid-base status should be evaluated, acidosis and ketosis may be present. Systolic arterial blood pressure should be measured, where hypovolaemic is suspected. Doppler measurement requires a 1- or 2-sized cuff (Critikon neonatal SOFT-CUF, GE Medical Systems, Information Technologies Gmbh, Freiburg, Germany) to be placed just proximal to the right elbow, ensuring cuff width was 50% of the circumference of this region. Conduction gel and the transducer are applied to the palmar distal, antebrachial surface, over the palmar common digital artery. Inflation of the cuff occludes the artery, then gradual deflation until the transducer detects the reentry of blood to the artery. The pressure measurement on the manometer correlates to systolic pressure. A mean of six readings should be used the reference range of 100–110 mm Hg, has been described in rabbits [41]. Following the same principles as used in cats and dogs, fluid therapy has been used to correct hypovolaemia in rabbits. Postsurgical adhesions have been minimized by the use of the calcium channel-blocking agent, verapamil (Verapamil, Securon) (200 µg/kg subcutaneously every 8 hours for 9 days) [42]. Analgesia, fluids, and nutritional support should be continued postoperatively. Prognosis is guarded to poor, as most rabbits have severe hepatic lipidosis, acidosis, ketosis, and severe gastric ulceration. Severe gastric ulceration could progress to perforation with subsequent peritonitis. Perforation carries a grave prognosis. Aggressive and early treatment will improve rate of recovery.

Gastric and intestinal neoplasia

Etiology

Neoplastic infiltrations including lymphoma, adenocarcinoma, leiomyo-sarcoma, and metastatic hemangiosarcoma have been reported as spontaneous neoplasms of the GIT in several breeds of rabbit [43]. There is a wide age range in reported cases, although juvenile and young adult rabbits appear to predominate.

Clinical features

Clinical signs seen with gastric tumors include anorexia, depression, appearance of cutaneous nodules (lymphoma), diarrhea, pallor, emaciation, and peripheral lymphadenopathy. Some rabbits may be asymptomatic until the disease is advanced and sudden death occurs. Duration of illness ranges from 1 week to 10 months [25,43–45].

Diagnosis

Iron-deficiency anemia without obvious blood loss suggests GIT bleeding, which may be caused by a tumor. Lymphoblastic leukemia, myeloid leukemia, lymphocytic leukemia with lymphocytosis including immature and typical lymphocytes, and an aleukemic picture with a relative lymphophilia, including immature and atypical lymphocytes have been described in rabbit lymphoma [44]. Plain and contrast imaging may reveal gastric wall thickening. Ultrasound-guided fine-needle aspiration of thickened lesions may produce cytologic preparations that are diagnostic. Although gastric endoscopy has the limitation of food and hair usually always being present in the rabbit stomach, some tumors may be obvious on endoscopy. In cases where only ulceration is seen, biopsy samples taken from the edge of the ulcer can be diagnostic for mucosal lymphoma.

Treatment and prognosis

Most cases of gastrointestinal adenocarcinoma are likely to be too advanced for surgical resection, and have a grave prognosis. Treatment protocols using alpha-interferon and isotretinoin proved unresponsive in rabbits with T-cell lymphoma [46]. Various chemotherapy and radiation therapy protocols described for cat or dog lymphoma could be extrapolated, especially as most chemotherapy drugs have been studied and used in experimental rabbits [3]. Prognosis would depend on stage of disease when diagnosed and response to therapy.

Gastric nematodes

Etiology

Obeliscoides cuniculi, a trichostrongyle, has been reported in North American domestic and wild rabbits. Transmission of nematodes is by fecal–oral ingestion of eggs, with subsequent migration of third-stage larvae that penetrate the gastric mucosa and develop into adults. The prepatent period is 16 to 20 days, and shedding continues for 61 to 118 days.

Clinical features

Although many rabbits are often asymptomatic, in heavy infestations anorexia, lethargy, and decreased weight gain may be seen.

Diagnosis

Eggs can be seen in fresh fecal smears or fecal flotation. A cobblestone, irregular, thickened appearance to the gastric mucosa and adult nematodes may be found on endoscopy or postmortem examination.

Treatment and prognosis

Ivermectin (Ivomec) (0.2–0.4 mg/kg subcutaneously, repeated in 10–14 days) is effective against *O cuniculi*. Prevention can then be achieved by feeding rabbits clean pasture products, uncontaminated by nematode eggs. Prognosis for recovery is good, unless the animal is severely stunted when treated, in which case it may never attain its anticipated body size.

Disorders of the intestinal tract

Bacterial enteritis

Clostridiosis and dysbiosis

Etiology. Clostridium spiroforme, Clostridium difficile, and *Clostridium perfringens* are bacteria associated with enteritis and enterotoxaemia in rabbits. Tyzzer's disease is caused by *Clostridium piliforme*. Clostridium organisms are widespread pathogenic bacteria, but also inhabit the adult rabbit GIT, along with Bacteroides, Enterococcus, Staphylococcus, Enterobacter, and *Escherichia coli*, as part of the normal intestinal flora [47]. Disease in adults is seen as a result of dysbiosis. Predisposing factors involved in cecal dysbiosis include sudden diet change altering pH and motility, stress causing immunosuppression and decreased GIT motility, or antibiotic administration, causing suppression of normal microbial flora. Bacteria such as *Bacteriodes*, are associated with exerting an inhibitory effect on potentially pathogenic bacteria including Clostridium and coliforms [48]. Mechanisms for antibiotic associated enteritis include: (1) alteration in intestinal motility and enterocyte ion transport was shown in lincomycin, clindamycin, erythromycin, and gentamicin [49,50]; and (2) altered microbial flora and overgrowth of *C difficile* and its cytotoxin following to oral ampicillin administration, and *C sporogenes* and its enterotoxin, following intravenous cephalosporin administration [51,52].

Disease in neonates and weanlings may be associated with high gastric pH 5 to 6.5, which allows clostridial proliferation and an underdeveloped population of normal GIT microbial flora. Young rabbits, 1 to 2 months old, have been shown to rely on interaction, with specific members of normal GIT microflora, between gut-associated lymphoid tissue and intestinal microflora, for antibody repertoire diversification [53]. Tyzzer's disease has been associated with the stress of overcrowding, unsanitary conditions, and concurrent disease.

Clinical features. Anorexia, depression, dehydration, hypothermia, intermittent or continuous diarrhea with hematochezia and mucus may be seen. In acute cases enterotoxic shock and death occurs within 24 to 48 hours. Chronic cases are occasionally seen with intermittent diarrhea and weight loss.

Diagnosis. Presumptive diagnosis is based on history of recent antibiotic administration, diet change, or stress. The clinical signs are not indicative of Clostridial diarrhea, and the spectrum of disease varies greatly. Isolation on culture is not diagnostic, as Clostridium species are part of the normal GIT microflora. Fecal *C perfringens* enterotoxin immunodetection is the most widely used diagnostic tool for *C perfringens* in both human beings and animals. Enzyme-linked immunoassay (ELISA) and latex agglutination assay are commercially available, although there are concerns about their sensitivities and specificities [54].

ELISA is also available for detection of *C difficile* toxin A and B; however, again, there are concerns about their specificities and sensitivities [54]. Detection of toxin B activity by the cell cytotoxicity assay is the current gold standard. Unfortunately, this assay requires up to 48 hours for confirmation of a negative result [55].

Treatment and prognosis. Aggressive fluid therapy and supportive therapy is essential in these critical patients. Cholestyramine (Questran) (2 g in 20 mL water, by gavage, every 24 hours) has been shown to bind to bacterial toxins, including clostridial cytotoxin and endotoxin in humans. Enteroxemia and mortality in rabbits, due to intravenous clindamycin, was prevented by cholestyramine administration on day 1 or 3 of the study [56]. Loperomide hydrochloride (Immodium) (0.1 mg/kg, oraly, every 8 hours for first 3 days, then every 24 hours for fourth and fifth days after the start of the diarrhea) [57] and a high-fiber diet may improve recovery. Prognosis for recovery of mild cases, that can be treated with diet adjustment can be good; however, severe cases have a poor prognosis.

Future treatments under current study include probiotics. There is an incomplete understanding of the mechanisms of probiotic activity; suggested mechanisms for reduction of pathogens include competition for nutrients, competition for enterocyte adhesion sites, and production of inhibitory substances [58]. Lactobacilli and enterococcus have been studied in rabbits. Lactobacilli, in contrast with other mammals, are very rarely found in the rabbit GIT microflora. Although some strains of lactobacilli, (*L fermentum*) were shown to have relatively resistant to pH 2 of rabbit gastric juice, lack of adhesive capability may prevent them colonizing the rabbit GIT [59]. *Enterococcus faecalis* and *Enterococcu faecuim*, the predominant enterococcal species in the rabbit GIT, were found in the feces of 8 of 10 healthy rabbits and in intestinal content of only 1 of 10. The enterococci were found to be resistant to a pH 3 broth, and transient inoculated enterococcal populations were demonstrated, suggesting colonization may occur, although further investigation is required [47]. Transfaunation of fresh caecotrophs from healthy rabbits can provide the appropriate microflora to help reestablish cecal homeostasis.

Coliobacillosis
Etiology. Severity of coliobacillosis presentation is variable, and is dependent on the particular strain of *E coli* [60] as well as on the presence of concurrent infectious agents [61]. Rabbit enteropathogenic *E coli* (rabbit EPEC or RDEC-1) strain is the most common cause of bacterial enteritis in rabbits. Rabbit EPEC is an attaching and effacing *E coli* strain, where bacterial adherence, via a fimbrial adhesin, results in destruction of the brush border and rearrangement of the enterocyte structure. High levels of Shiga toxin are not expressed by EPEC strains [62]. Transmission is by the fecal–oral route.

Clinical features. Neonates, 1 to 14 days old, or young rabbits, 2 to 4 months old, stressed by weaning, transport, or over crowding, are most likely to show clinical signs. Clinical signs include acute diarrhea, weight loss, intussusception, and rectal prolapse, with mortality rates ranging between 50% to 100%.

Diagnosis. Presumptive diagnosis can be made on isolation of *E coli* in feces of affected animals, although dysbiosis often causes proliferation of nonpathogenic *E coli*. Definitive diagnosis is based on histopathologic identification of *E coli* attachment to enterocytes.

Treatment and prognosis. Broad-spectrum antibiotics such as enrofloxacin or once hydrated trimethoprim-suphadoxine (Delvoprim Coject) (48 mg/kg subcutaneously, every 24 hours), Trimethoprim–sulfamethoxazole (Cotrimoxazole suspension) (30 mg/kg orally, every 12 hours) should be started while awaiting culture and sensitivity. Early, aggressive fluid therapy and supportive treatment is essential to optimize a successful outcome. Loperamide hydrochloride and fluid rehydration proved successful in the treatment of an *E coli* outbreak in 22 adult New Zealand white rabbits all fully recovered within 2 weeks [57]. Prognosis is guarded to poor, but is dependent on the strain of *E coli*, immunocompetence of the animal and presence of synergistic copathogens such as *Lawsonia intracellularis* (Campylobacter-like organism) or *rotavirus* [62].

Miscellaneous bacteria

Etiology. Salmonella and pseudomonas species, *Yersinia pseudotuberculosis* and *L intracellularis* may cause acute or chronic enterocolitis in rabbits. Neonates and weanling rabbits are most severely affected, with variable morbidity and mortality rates. Transmission is by the fecal–oral route, contaminated feed or water. Zoonotic potential exists.

Clinical features. Salmonellosis and acute *Y pseudotuberculosis* rapidly progresses to septicemia and death. Chronic *Y pseudotuberculosis* is associated with diarrhea and visceral and mesenteric microabscess formation. Low morbidity, high mortality rates have been seen with *Pseudomonas aeruginosa*.

Diagnosis. In cases where these bacteria are suspected, the laboratory must be informed as specific enrichment, and selection procedures are recommended for the culture and sensitivity of these organisms.

Treatment and prognosis. Treatment is supportive, with antibiosis based on culture and sensitivity. Prognosis is uncertain, but seems to be good if the bacteria can identified by culture and treated early and aggressively.

Viral enteritis

Etiology

Viral enteritis is primarily seen in young, weanling rabbits, with rotavirus affecting 30- to 80-day-old rabbits and coronavirus affecting 21- to 70-day-old rabbits. Rotaviral maternal antibodies fall to undetectable levels at day 60, while antibody production by the affected rabbit occurs between 45 to 60 days [63]. The trough in antibody level is the point of rotavirus and infection, maximum viral shedding, and rapid antibody production. Transmission is airborne and fecal–oral. Viral infection causes villous atrophy with lymphocytic inflammation, particularly in the ileum and intestinal distension. Coronavirus has also been associated with cardiomyopathy and pleural infusion.

Clinical features. Maternal antibody for rotavirus can provide some protection, resulting in subclinical shedding of virus for about three days. Soft feces to diarrhea are often the main clinical sign of rotavirus infection. However coinfection with *E coli* was shown to result in increased mortality (50–80%) due to diarrheal disease compared with *E coli* alone [61].

High morbidity and mortality is associated with coronavirus; 100% mortality was seen in an outbreak within 24 hours of onset of clinical signs. Clinical signs include diarrhea, abdominal distension, and lethargy [64].

Diagnosis. Diagnosis of rotavirus is on virus isolation, antibody detection, or histopathology.

A definitive diagnosis of coronavirus can be made on histopathology or virus isolation in the feces. Virus can be found in clinically normal adult rabbits.

Treatment and prognosis. Supportive treatment of rotavirus infection is usually successful, except in cases of simultaneous coinfection with another enteropathogen, which carries a guarded prognosis. Coronavirus enteritis has a guarded to poor prognosis.

Parasitic enteritis

Nematodes, cestodes, and trematodes
Etiology. Passalurus ambiguus, the pinworm, is common in domestic rabbits and widespread in wild rabbits. Transmission of embryonated ova is by fecal–oral. Adult worms, 2 to 11 mm long, inhabit the cecum and colon, and are often seen when they are passed in fresh feces [65]. *Graphidium stringosum, Trichostrongylus retortaeformis,* and *calcaratus* are nematodes found commonly in wild rabbits in Europe and North America, and infections may be found in domestic rabbits allowed to graze infected pasture.

The rabbit is the intermediate host for several tapeworms that affect dogs and foxes including *Cysticercus pisiformis,* the larval stage of *Taenia pisiformis, Coenurus serialis,* the larval stage of *Taenia serialis,* and *Echinococcus granulosus.* Transmission is by fecal–oral ingestion of eggs, shed in carnivore feces. Larvae migrate from the intestines to the liver, lung, lymph nodes, intermuscular connective tissue, and occasionally the orbit or brain, depending on their predilection site. The rabbit is one of the primary hosts for *Cittotaenia variables,* where the oribatid mite may be the intermediate host.

Clinical features. Although reported to be nonpathogenic, peri-anal pruritus may be seen in heavy infections. Studies of *P ambiguus* in the wild suggests no acquired resistance in rabbits [66].

Cestode infection is usually asymptomatic, but in heavy infestations abdominal distension, lethargy, and weight loss may be seen. *C serialis* usually form subcutaneous cysts, palpated as soft tissue swellings, although cysts can occur at any of their predilection sites. Clinical signs will be depend on the site and extent of the space-occupying lesion.

Diagnosis. P ambiguus ova are intermittently shed and can be found on fecal flotation or fresh fecal smears, where adult worms may also be identified.

Definitive diagnosis of tapeworm larvae can be made on examination of tissue biopsy or fluid aspiration of cysts.

Treatment and prognosis. Various anthelmintics are effective against *P ambiguus,* Fenbendazole (Panacur) (10–20 mg/kg, repeated in 10–14 days), thiabendazole (Thiabendazole) (50 mg/kg orally, repeated in 10–14 days) are effective against this parasite. However, ivermectin (Ivomec) was shown to be ineffective against *P ambiguus* in studies using doses of 0.4, 1.0, and 2.0 mg/kg injected subcutaneously [67]. Prognosis of a full recovery is good; however, prevention and eradication of *P ambiguus* can be extremely difficult, as the pinworm ova are relatively resistant to heat and a wide variety of disinfectants.

Praziquantel (Droncit) (5–10 mg/kg orally, single dose) is recommended in the treatment of cestodes and trematodes. *T serialis* cysts should ideally be surgically excised or drained by aspiration. Prognosis of recovery is good, unless the animal is severely affected by the space-occupying lesion or liver pathology. Prevention can be achieved by avoiding carnivore feces-contaminated grass.

Cryptosporidiosis

Etiology. Cryptosporidiosis is caused by *Cryptosporidium parvum*. Rabbits become infested when they ingest the sporulated oocysts, which are shed in feces, but may be transmitted in water, fomites, or contaminated feed. The prepatent period is 3 to 21 days.

Clinical features. Adult rabbits tend to be subclinical or asymptomatic, unless immunocompromised. Neonate or young rabbits stressed by weaning, transport, or over crowding are most likely to show clinical signs. Lethargy, poor body condition and coat quality, decreased appetite, dehydration, weight loss, and pasty, unformed feces to diarrhea lasting 3 to 5 days, have been reported in natural and experimental infections [65,68]. Neonates were found to have variably severe, transient infection, present from 3 to 21 days postinfection. Villous blunting and eosinophilic inflammation of the lamina propria of the entire GIT, was found in experimental infection of neonate (3-day-old) rabbits. No histologic evidence of infection was found in the adult (180-day-old) rabbits also examined in the study.

Diagnosis. Diagnosis requires finding the oocysts on fecal examination. Magnification ×1000 is required, as *C parvum* is the smallest of the coccidians. Use of immunofluorescence and acid-fast stains improves sensitivity [14].

Treatment and prognosis. Currently, there are no known reliable treatments. Prognosis of recovery is guarded to good, depending on the severity of infection and degree of villous blunting. Severely stunted rabbits may never attain its anticipated body size.

Intestinal coccidiosis

Etiology. Many different species of Eimeria have been identified in the rabbit. With predominance of *Eimeria perforans*, *E media*, and *E magna* in domestic breeding colonies wide spread, and *E perforans* is most common in wild rabbits in France and Australia [69]. Transmission is by ingestion of sporulated oocysts. It is generally accepted that caecotrophy is not involved in the transmission of infectious oocysts. Prepatent periods for the *Eimeria* species range from 2 to 10 days, and sporulation requires 22 hours at 20°C for *E perforans* and 70 hours for *E piriformis* [65].

Clinical features. Intestinal coccidiosis is most often a subclinical disease in adult immunocompetent rabbits. Coinfection with other enteropathies, immunosuppression or a naive immune system, dose of infection, and species of Eimeria are all predisposing factors to clinical disease. Clinical signs include: weight loss, mild to severe intermittent or continuous hemorrhagic diarrhea, dehydration, and occasionally intussusceptions. Death is usually associated with secondary bacterial enteritis and dehydration. A 4.5-cm ileo-ileal intussusception was diagnosed, in a 14-week-old rabbit, suspected consequent to hyperperistalsis induced by *E perforans* infection [70].

Diagnosis. Coccidiosis is presumptively diagnosed by finding oocysts on fecal flotation. Even on repeated fecal examination, small numbers of oocysts does not determine their clinical significance. Definitive diagnosis is based on histopathologic findings (Fig. 5).

Treatment and prognosis. Trimethoprim–sulfamethoxazole (Co-trimoxazole suspension) (30 mg/kg orally, every 12 hours for 10 days) has been shown to be effective. Prognosis is good in mild cases, and may result in lifelong immunity.

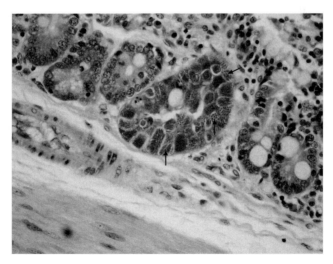

Fig. 5. Photomicrograph of small intestinal epithelium of a rabbit with coccidiosis. Prominent intraepithelial coccidial schizonts can be seen (*arrows*). (Courtesy of M.J. Day, BVMS (Hons), PhD, DECVP, FRCPath, FRCVS, University of Bristol.)

Mucoid enteropathy (rabbit epizootic enteropathy)

Etiology

Mucoid enteropathy is an idiopathic, widespread condition resulting in goblet cell hyperplasia and excessive mucous production within the intestinal tract. Mucoid enteropathy is mainly seen in young rabbits of 4- to 14-week-old rabbits, although there have been reports of older rabbits, for example, 7 months old [71]. Mucoid enteropathy may occur concurrent with other enteropathies. Lesions of mucoid enteropathy have been found associated with cecal hyperacidity due to abnormal volatile fatty acid production or absorption and dysbiosis [72], fiber-deficient diet [73], and dysautonomia [74].

Clinical features. Associated clinical signs that have been reported, include anorexia, depression, abdominal pain and distention, weight loss, dehydration, hypothermia, diarrhea initially, progressing to mucus excretion, or constipation and palpation of a firm, dough-like, large cecum. Acute mortality can occur within 1 to 3 days, reaching rates of 30% to 80%, and chronic disease with mortality may occur within 7 to 9 days [65,75].

Diagnosis. Presumptive diagnosis can be made on history and clinical signs, although may mimic other enteropathies. Radiography may show evidence of cecal impaction, and in later cases evidence of gastric and intestinal stasis. Definitive diagnosis is on postmortem findings of copious intestinal mucous and goblet cell hyperplasia (Fig. 6).

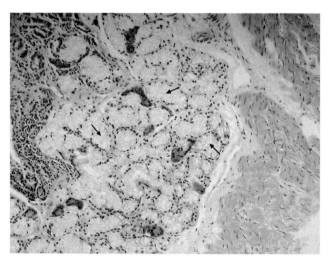

Fig. 6. Photomicrograph colonic epithelium of a rabbit with mucoid enteropathy. Prominent goblet cell hyperplasia (*arrows*). (Courtesy of R. Cecchi, MVB, MSc, MRCVS and G.R. Pearson, BVMS, PhD, FRCPath, MRCVS, University of Bristol.)

Treatment and prognosis. Nonspecific supportive treatment is recommended. In cases of constipation the use of frequent enemas has been described [76]. Prognosis is poor. Prevention can be achieved by feeding a high-fiber, low-carbohydrate diet [73].

Dysautonomia and cecal impaction

Etiology

Dysautonomia in the rabbit is an idiopathic condition that causes loss of autonomic nervous system function. Twenty rabbits with clinical signs of mucoid enteropathy were later confirmed on postmortem examination to be dysautonomia [77]. Further research into the early stages of mucoid enteropathy makes it a good model for the study of dysautonomia [74].

Clinical features. Dysautonomia is associated with clinical signs of gastrointestinal stasis and autonomic nerve deficits. Symptoms include dry mucous membranes and conjunctiva, dilated pupils, bradycardia, urine retention and overflow incontinence, dilated, firm, impacted colon, proprioceptive deficits, and loss of anal tone. Accumulation of food in mouth and dysphagia and evidence of lower respiratory disease due to aspiration pneumonia, secondary to dysphagia and megaoesophagus may also be seen. This condition is associated with a high mortality in all affected species.

Diagnosis. A presumptive diagnosis can be made on clinical signs. Radiography of the thorax and abdomen may reveal evidence of aspiration pneumonia, megaoesophagus, impacted colon, and a large bladder. Absent tear production can be demonstrated with a Schirmer tear test, average tear production in rabbits is 5 mm/min $\pm$ 2.4mm/min [78]. Dramatic miosis within 45 minutes occurs in dogs in response to diluted (0.1%) pilocarpine (Pilocarpine), due to denervation hypersensitivity.

Definitive diagnosis requires demonstration of the characteristic lesions of chromolytic degeneration of autonomic neurons, found on histology and electron microscopy, similar to equine grass sickness and feline and hare dysautonomias, at postmortem examination.

Treatment and prognosis. Supportive treatment includes fluid therapy, force feeding, eye lubrication, enemas, and bladder emptying. Bethanechol (Myotonine; 0.04 mg/kg) enables many affected cats and dogs to void urine normally and completely. Prognosis is poor, although in other species some animals have spontaneously recovered.

Anorectal papilloma

Etiology and clinical features

Anorectal papillomas are small friable, fungating masses, originate from the rectal squamous columnar epithelium, at the anorectal junction. These benign tumors are well differentiated and are not related to viral papillomas of the skin and oral cavity. Some rabbits are asymptomatic, clinical signs include constipation, discomfort, hemorrhage from the anus, and in severe cases, rectal prolapse.

Diagnosis. A presumptive diagnosis is usually made on clinical features; however, excisional biopsy and histopathology is required fro a definitive diagnosis.

Treatment and prognosis. Surgical excision is curative provided all of the abnormal tissue is removed. In asymptomatic cases, spontaneous regression can occur; prognosis for full recovery is good.

Summary

The gastrointestinal tract is a common site of disease in the rabbit. Diet-related disease and stress-related disease predominate and can play a large role in preventative medicine. However, bacterial, viral, parasitic, idiopathic, and neoplastic diseases are also seen frequently in the pet rabbit.

References

[1] Walberg J. Osteogenic sarcoma with metastasis in a rabbit (*Orycytolagus cuniculus*). Lab Anim Sci 1981;31(4):407–8.
[2] Redrobe S. Surgical procedures and dental disorders. In: Flecknell PA, editor. BSAVA manual of rabbit medicine and surgery. Gloucester: British Small Animal Association; 2000. p. 117–40.
[3] Heatley JJ, Smith AN. Spontaneous neoplasms of lagomorphs. Exotic Anim Clin North Am 2004;7:561–77.
[4] Weisman DL, Olmstead ML, Kowalski JJ. In vitro evaluation of antibiotic elution from polymethylmethacrylate (PMMA) and mechanical assessment of antibiotic–PMMA composites. Vet Surg 2000;29(3):245–51.
[5] Ethell MT, Bennett RA, Brown MP, et al. In vitro elution of gentamicin, amikacin, and ceftiofur from polymethylmethacrylate and hydroxyapatite cement. Vet Surg 2000;29(5): 375–82.
[6] Straw RC, Powers BE, Klausner J, et al. Canine mandibular osteosarcoma: 51 cases (1980–1992). J Am Anim Hosp Assoc 1996;32(2):257–62.
[7] Salm R, Field J. Osteosarcoma in a rabbit. J Pathol Bacteriol 1965;89(89):400–2.
[8] Hoover J, Paulsen D, Qualls C, et al. Osteosarcoma with subcutaneous involvement in a rabbit. J Am Vet Med Assoc 1968;189:1156–8.
[9] Weisbroth S, Hurvitz A. Spontaneous osteogenic sarcoma in *Orcytolagus cuniculus* with elevated serum alkaline phosphatase. Lab Anim Care 1969;19:263–6.
[10] Sunderberg JP, Junge RE, El Schazly MO. Oral papillomatosis in New Zealand white rabbits. Am J Vet Res 1985;46(3):664–8.
[11] Dominguez JA, Corella EL, Auro A. Oral papillomatosis in two laboratory rabbits in Mexico. Lab Anim Sci 1981;31:71–3.
[12] Weisbroth SH, Scher S. Spontaneous oral papillomatosis in rabbits. J Am Vet Med Assoc 1970;157:1940–4.

[13] Embers ME, Budgeon LR, Pickel M, et al. Protective immunity to rabbit oral and cutaneous papillomaviruses by immunization with short peptides of L2, the minor capsid protein. J Virol 2002;76(19):9798–805.

[14] Willard MD. The digestive system. In: Nelson RE, Couto GC, editors. Small animal internal medicine. Volume 3. St. Louis (MO): Mosby; 2003. p. 415, 447.

[15] Cruise LJ, Brewer NR. Anatomy. In: Manning PJ, Ringler DH, Newcomer CE, editors. The biology of the laboratory rabbit. Volume 2. San Diego (CA): Academic; 1994. p. 47–61.

[16] Leary SL, Manning PJ, Anderson LC. Experimental and naturally-occurring gastric foreign bodies in laboratory rabbits. Lab Anim Sci 1984;34(1):58–61.

[17] Deeb B. Digestive system and disorders. In: Flecknell PA, editor. BSAVA manual of rabbit medicine and surgery. Gloucester: British Small Animal Veterinary Association; 2000. p. 39–46.

[18] Lanas A, Royo Y, Ortego J, et al. Experimental esophagitis induced by acid pepsin in rabbits mimicking human reflux esophagitis. Gastroenterology 1999;116:97–107.

[19] Wright H, Kieffer CA, Dinda PK, et al. Mechanisms of rabbit esophageal mucosal resistance to acid injury [abstract]. Gastroenterology 1995;108(4):A260.

[20] Kounenis G, Koutsoviti-Papadopoulou M, Elezoglou A, et al. Comparative study of the H2-receptor antagonists Cimetodine, Ranitidine, Famotidine and Nizatidine on the rabbit stomach fundus and sigmoid colon. J Pharmacobiodyn 1992;15:561–5.

[21] Hinton M. Gastric ulceration in the rabbit. J Comp Pathol 1980;90(3):475–81.

[22] Man WK, Silcocks PB, Waldes R, et al. Histology of experimental stress ulcer: the effect of cimetidine on adrenaline gastric lesions in the rabbit. Br J Exp Pathol 1981;62(4):411–8.

[23] Collin BJ. Stress ulcer induced by hypovolemic shock in female rabbit. Anat Histiol Emryol Zentral Vet 1977;6(1):94.

[24] Manekar MS, Waghmare ML. Pharmacological study of aspirin induced acute gastric ulceration in rabbits [abstract]. Indian J Med Res 1980;71:926–32.

[25] Gupta BN. Lymphosarcoma in a rabbit. Am J Vet Res 1976;37:841–3.

[26] Redfern JS, Lin HJ, McArthur KE, et al. Gastric-acid and pepsin hypersecretion in conscious rabbits. Am J Physiol 1991;261(2):G295–304.

[27] Meredith A. Ileus and the obstructed rabbit. Paper presented at the BSAVA Congress, Scientific proceedings, Birmingham; 2002. p. 353–4.

[28] Parga ML. Assessment of the efficacy of meloxicam and development of a pain scoring system based on behaviour in rabbits undergoing elective surgery. Paper presented at the British Small Animal Veterinary Association 46th Annual Congress, Birmingham; 2003. p. 555.

[29] Michiels M, Monbaliu J, Hendricks R, et al. Pharmakokinetics and tissue distribution of the new gastrokinetic agent cisapride in rat, rabbit and dog. Arzneimittelforschung 1987; 37(10):1159–67.

[30] Gintant GA, Limberis JT, McDermott JS, et al. The canine purkinje fibre: an in vitro model system for acquired long QT syndrome and drug-induced delayed repolarization and prolongation of the QT interval. J Cardiovasc Pharmacol 2001;37(5):607–18.

[31] Washabau RJ. Gastrointestinal motility disorders and gastrointestinal prokinetic therapy. Small Anim Clin North Am 2003;33:1007–28.

[32] Drici MD, Edert SN, Wang WX, et al. Comparison of tegaserod (HTF 919) and its main human metabolite with cisaride and erythromycin on cardiac repolarization in the isolated rabbit heart. J Cardiovasc Pharmacol 1999;34(1):82–8.

[33] Wiseman LR, Faulds D. Cisapride—an updated review of its pharmacology and therapeutic efficacy as a prokinetic agent in gastrointestinal motility disorders. Drugs 1994;47(1):116–52.

[34] Kitazawa T, Ichikawa S, Yokoyama T, et al. Stimulating action of KW-5139 (Leu (13)-Motilin) on gastrointestinal motiliy in the rabbit. Br J Pharmacol 1994;111(1):288–94.

[35] Baldazzi C, Barbanti M, Basaglia R, et al. A new series of 6-chloro-2,3-dihydro-4(1H)-quinazolinone derviatives as antiemetic and gastrointestinal motility enhancing agents. Arzneimittelforschung 1996;46(9):911–8.

[36] Sato F, Sekiguchi M, Marui S, et al. EM574, an erythromycin derivative, is a motilin receptor agonist in the rabbit. Eur J Pharmacol 1997;322:63–71.

[37] Rogers G, Taylor C, Austin JC, et al. A pharngostomy technique for chronic oral dosing of rabbits. Lab Anim Sci 1988;38(5):619–20.

[38] Smith DA, Olson PO, Mathews KA. Nutritional support for rabbits using the percutaneously placed gastrotomy tube: a preliminary study. J Am Anim Hosp Assoc 1997;33:48–54.

[39] Gillett NA, Brooks DL, Tillman PC. Medical and surgical management of gastric obstruction from a hairball in the rabbit. J Am Vet Med Assoc 1983;183(11):1176–8.

[40] Wilson RB, Holscher MA, Sly DL. Liver lobe torsion in a rabbit. Lab Anim Sci 1987;37(4): 506–7.

[41] Erhart W, Henke J. Essential facts of blood in dogs and cats. 3rd edition. Babenhausen, Germany: Vet Verlag; 2003.

[42] Steinleitner A, Lambert H, Kazensky C, et al. Reduction of primary postoperative adhesion formation under calcium blockade in the rabbit. J Surg Res 1990;48:42–5.

[43] Shibuya K, Tajima M, Kanai K, et al. Spontaneous lymphoma in a Japanese White Rabbit. J Vet Med Sci 1999;61(12):1327–9.

[44] Toth LA, Olson GA, Wilson E, et al. Lymphocytic leukemia and lymphosarcoma in a rabbit. J Am Vet Med Assoc 1990;197(5):627–9.

[45] Gómez A, Gázquez V, Roncero C, et al. Lymphoma in a rabbit: histopathological and immunohistochemical findings. J Small Anim Pract 2002;43:224–6.

[46] White S, Campbell T, Logan A, et al. Lymphoma with cutaneous involvement in three domestic rabbits (Orycytolagus cuniculus). Vet Dermatol 2000;11:61–7.

[47] Linaje R, Coloma MD, Pérez-Martínez G, et al. Characterization of faecal enterococci from rabbits for the selection of probiotic strains. J Appl Microbiol 2004;96:761–71.

[48] Fesce A, Ceccarelli A, Fesce E, et al. Ecophylaxis: preventative treatment with gentimicin of rabbit lincomycin-associated diarrhea. Folia Vet Lat 1977;7(3):225–42.

[49] Goldhill JM, Rose K, Percy WH. Effects of antibiotics on epithelial ion transport in the rabbit distal colon in vitro. J Pharm Pharmacol 1996;48(6):651–6.

[50] Navarro H, Arruebo MP, Alcalde AI, et al. Effect of erythromycin on D-galactose absorption and sucrase activity in the rabbit jejunum. Can J Physiol Pharmacol 1993; 71(3–4):191–4.

[51] Guandalini S, Fassano A, Migliavacca M, et al. Pathogenesis of postantibiotic diarrhoea caused by Clostridium difficile: an in vitro study in the rabbit intestine. Gut 1988;29(5): 598–602.

[52] Hara-Kudo Y, Morishita Y, Nagaoka Y, et al. Incidence of diarrhea with antibiotics and the increase of clostridia in rabbits. J Vet Med Sci 1996;58(12):1181–5.

[53] Lanning D, Sethupathi P, Rhee K, et al. Intestinal microflora and diversification of the rabbit antibody repertoire. J Immunol 2000;165:2012–9.

[54] Marks SL, Kather EJ. Bacterial-associated diarrhea in the dog: a critical appraisal. Small Anim Vet Clin North Am 2003;33:1029–60.

[55] Landry ML, Topal J, Ferguson D, et al. Evaluation of biosite triage Clostridium difficile panel for rapid detection of Clostridium difficile in stool samples. J Clin Microbiol 2001;39(5): 1855–8.

[56] Lipman NS, Weischedel AK, Connors MJ, et al. Utilization of cholestyramine resin as preventative treatment for antibiotic (clindamycin) induced enterotoxaemia in the rabbit. Lab Anim 1992;26:1–8.

[57] Banerjee AK, Angulo AF, Dhasmana KM, et al. Acute diarrhoeal disease in the rabbit: bacteriological diagnosis and efficacy of oral rehydration in combination with loperamide hydrochloride. Lab Anim 1987;21:314–7.

[58] Moore J. The use of probiotics in the calf: An overview. Br Cattle Vet Assoc 2004;12(2): 125–8.

[59] Yu B, Tsen HY. Lactobacillus cells in the rabbit digestive tract and the factors affecting their distribution. J Appl Bacteriol 1993;75:269–75.

[60] Peeters JE, Geeroms R, Orskov F. Biotype, serotype, and pathogenicity of attaching and effacing enteropathogenic *Escherichia coli* strains isolated from diarrheic commercial rabbits. Infect Immunol 1988;56:1442–8.

[61] Thouless ME, DiGiacomo RF, Deeb BJ. The effect of combined Rotavirus and *Escherichia coli* infections in rabbits. Lab Anim Sci 1996;46(4):381–5.

[62] Schauer DB, McCathey SN, Daft BM, et al. Proliferative enterocolitis associated with dual infection with enteropathogenic *Escherichia coli* and *Lawsonia intracellularis* in rabbits. J Clin Microbiol 1998;36(6):1700–3.

[63] DiGiacomo RF, Thouless ME. Age-related antibodies to Rotavirus in New Zealand rabbits. J Clin Microbiol 1984;19(5):710–1.

[64] DiGiacomo RF, Mare CJ. Viral diseases. In: Manning PJ, Ringler DH, Newcomer CE, editors. The biology of the laboratory rabbit. 2nd edition. San Diego: Academic Press; 1994. p. 171–204.

[65] Harkness JE, Wagner JE. Specific diseases and conditions. Biology and medicine of rabbits and rodents. 4th edition. Philadelphia: Williams & Wilkins; 1995. p. 262.

[66] Boag B. The incidence of helminth parasites from the wild rabbit *Orcytolagus cuniculus* (L.) in Eastern Scotland. J Helminthol 1985;59:61–9.

[67] Tsui TLH, Patton NM. Comparative efficacy of subcutaneous injection doses of ivermectin against P. ambiguus in rabbits. J Appl Rabbit Res 1991;14:266–9.

[68] Mosier DA, Cimon KY, Kuhls TL, et al. Experimental cryptosporidiosis in adult and neonatal rabbits. Vet Parasitol 1997;69:163–9.

[69] Voza GV, Chabaud A, Landau I. Coccidiosis of the wild rabbit (*Orycytolagus cuniculus*) in France. Parasite 2003;10:51–7.

[70] Weisbroth SH, Scher S. Fatal intussusception associated with intestinal coccidiosis (*Eimeria perforans*) in a rabbit. Lab Anim Sci 1975;25(1):79–81.

[71] Vandekerchove D, Roels S, Charlier G. A naturally occurring case of Epizootic enteropathy in a specific-pathogen-free rabbit colony. Vlaams Diergeneeskundig Tijdschrift 2001;70: 486–90.

[72] Lelkes L, Chang C. Microbial dysbiosis in rabbit mucoid enteropathy. Lab Anim Sci 1987; 37(6):757–64.

[73] Bernhardt W. Ein Beitrag zur Ätiologie, Prophylaxe und therapie der Enteropathia mucinosa beim Hauskanninchen. Monateshefte Vet 1992;47(3):149–53.

[74] Whitwell K, Needham J. Mucoid enteropathy in UK rabbits: dysautonomia confirmed. Vet Rec 1996;139:323–4.

[75] Marlier D, Vindevogel H. L'entérocolite epizootique du lapin. Ann Med Vet 1998;142: 281–4.

[76] Breitweiser B. Mucoid enteropathy in rabbits. Presented at the Proceedings of the North American Vet Conference, Orlando, FL, January, 1997. p. 782–3.

[77] Van Der Hage M, Dorrestein GM. Caecal impaction in the rabbit: relationship with dysautonomia. Paper presented at the 6th World Rabbit Congress Lempedes, France; 1996. p. 77–80.

[78] Abrams KL, Brooks DE, Funk RS, et al. Evaluation of the Schirmer tear test in clinically normal rabbits. Am J Vet Res 1990;51:1912–3.

ELSEVIER
SAUNDERS

Vet Clin Exot Anim 8 (2005) 377–391

VETERINARY
CLINICS
Exotic Animal Practice

Index

Note: Page numbers of article titles are in **boldface** type.

A

Abdominal distention, in piscine gastroenterology, 248–249

Abscesses, periapical, in rabbits, 342

Acid-fast staining, for amphibian gastroenterology, 225, 230–231
  for piscine gastroenterology, 251–252
  for rabbit gastroenterology, 358

Acid-peptic disorders, in human gastroenterology, 178–181

Acid secretion, gastrointestinal, in ferrets, 189–190

Adenocarcinoma, in ferrets, 209
  in rabbits, 352

Adenomas, in amphibians, 231
  in ferrets, colonic, 209

Adenovirus(es), in raptors, 310–311
  in reptiles, gastrointestinal, 279–280

Aerobic bacteria, in cloaca, of raptors, 303

Amphibian gastroenterology, **217–235**
  anatomy for, 217–221
    of adults, 218–221
    of larvae, 217–218
  bacterial enteritis, 231
  clinical disease signs, 221–223
    in adults, 222–223
    in larvae, 221–222
  cloacal prolapse, 228–229
  common diseases, 226–232
    in adults, 226–232
    in larvae, 226
  diagnostic methods for, 223–226
    blood work, 224
    cytology/histology, 225–226, 230–231
    endoscopy, 225
    fecal examination, 223–224
    imaging, 224–225
  emergency management of, 226, 228
  food impaction, 228
  foreign object ingestion, 228
  granulomatous conditions, 229–230
  intussusception, 229
  neoplasia, 231
  nutritional disorders, 231
  orders included in, 217
  parasitism, 223–224, 227
  physiology for, 217–221
    of adults, 218–221
    of larvae, 217–218
  treatment options, 226–232
    in adults, 226–232
    in larvae, 226
  viral enteritis, 231

Amphotericin B, for *M ornithogaster* infection, 290, 294–295
  in psittacines, 331

Anaerobic bacteria, facultative. See *Macrohabdus ornithogaster.*
  in psittacine gastroenterology, 330–331, 335

Anamnesis, in reptile gastroenterology, 272

Anorectal papilloma, in rabbits, 361–362

Anorexia, in amphibians, 222, 231
  in ferrets, 204, 206
  in piscines, 249

Antemortem detection, of *M ornithogaster*, 292–293

Anti-inflammatory drugs, in ferret gastroenterology, 213
  in human gastroenterology, 181
    avian applications of, 183
  in psittacine gastroenterology, 330

Antibiotics, for *M ornithogaster*, 289–290
  in ferret gastroenterology, 183–184, 213
    for *H mustelae* infections, 198, 200
  in human gastroenterology, 180–181
    ferret applications of, 183–184
  in piscine gastroenterology, 252, 255
  in psittacine gastroenterology, 330–331

Antibody detection, with ferret infections,
    of *H mustelae,* 192–193, 196
    viral, 207

Antifungal agents, for candidiasis, in
    raptors, 306

Antigen detection, for infection diagnosis,
    avian applications of, 182
        ferret applications of, 183–184
        in human gastroenterology,
            174–175

Anus, in piscines, 243

Ascarid infestations, in reptiles, 285

Ascites, in amphibians, 222
    in piscines, 249

Autoantibodies, with *H mustelae* infections,
    in ferrets, 192–193, 196

Autoimmune disease, markers of, in human
    gastroenterology, 175

Avian poxvirus, in psittacines, 323–324

Avian species, gastrointestinal tract
    disorders of, challenges with, 181–182
        human gastroenterology
            applications for, 182–183
        psittacine, **319–339.** See also
            Psittacine gastroenterology.
        raptor, **297–317.** See also *Raptor
            gastroenterology.*
    M ornithogaster infections of, 290–292

B

Bacteria, aerobic, in raptor cloaca, 303
    anaerobic, in psittacine
        gastroenterology, 330–331, 335
    facultative anaerobic. See
        Macrohabdus ornithogaster.

Bacterial infections, gastrointestinal, in
    amphibians, 231
        in ferrets, 204–207
        in humans, 175, 183
        in piscines, 251–253
        in psittacines, 335
        in rabbits, 183, 353–356
        in reptiles, 280–281

Beak, in amphibian larvae, anatomy of,
    217–218
    in raptors, anatomy of, 299
        disorders of, 304–305, 307

Behavioral history, in piscine
    gastroenterology, 247

Biliary system. See *Hepatobiliary system.*

Biochemical profiles. See *Laboratory tests.*

Biopsy(ies), in ferret gastroenterology, 184,
    204–205, 207–208, 211–212
        for *H mustelae,* 194–196
    in human gastroenterology, 175, 184
    in psittacine gastroenterology, 328,
        330
    in rabbit gastroenterology, 343–344

Birds. See *Avian species.*

Blood chemistry screens, in ferret
    gastroenterology, 210
    in piscine gastroenterology, 248

Blood cultures, for *H mustelae,* in ferrets,
    195

Blood work. See *Laboratory tests.*

Bone disease, metabolic, in amphibians, 232

Breeding techniques, for *M ornithogaster*
    elimination, 295

Burns, esophageal, in psittacines, 327

C

Calcium disorders, in amphibians, 232

Campylobacter jejuni, in ferret
    gastroenterology, 204–207

Candidiasis, in psittacines, 325
    in raptors, 306

Canine distemper virus (CDV), in ferrets,
    gastrointestinal, 205–207

Capillaria infections, gastrointestinal, in
    raptors, 306–307

Capsule endoscopy, in human
    gastroenterology, 176–180
        avian applications of, 182
        ferret applications of, 184

Catfish, enteric septicemia of, 255

Ceca, impaction of, in rabbits, 361
    in raptors, anatomy of, 301–303
    paired, in psittacines, 322

Cells of Ito, in piscines, 245

Cestode infestations, in amphibians, 227
    in piscines, 256
    in rabbits, 357–358
    in reptiles, 284

Chelating agents, for heavy metal toxicosis,
    in psittacines, 332
        in reptiles, 274

Cholecystokinin, in ferret gastroenterology,
    176

Chromomycosis, in amphibians, 229–230

Chyme, in psittacines, 322–323

Circulatory shock, in amphibians, 222

Cloaca, of amphibians, disorders of, 223, 228–229
  of piscine, anatomy of, 243
    disorders of, 249–250
  of psittacines, anatomy of, 322–323
    disorders of, 335–336
  of raptors, anatomy of, 301, 303
  of reptiles, anatomy of, 271
    disorders of, 285

Cloacal lavage, in piscine gastroenterology, 249–250

Cloacal prolapse, in amphibians, 223, 228–229
  in psittacines, 335–336
  in reptiles, 285

Clostridiosis, in rabbits, 353–355

Clostridium enteritis, in psittacines, 335
  in rabbits, 183

Coccidiosis, intestinal, in ferrets, 205–206
  in piscines, 254–255
  in rabbits, 359
  in reptiles, 282–283

Coelomic endoscopy, for amphibian gastroenterology, 225

Coelomic swelling, in amphibians, 222, 228

Coliobacillosis, in rabbits, 355

Colon, of ferrets, 190
  adenomas of, 209
  of psittacines, 322–323
  of raptors, anatomy of, 301, 303
  of reptiles, anatomy of, 270

Complete blood count, in ferret gastroenterology, 210
  in piscine gastroenterology, 248

Computed tomography (CT) scan, for amphibian gastroenterology, 225
  for human gastroenterology, 178
    avian applications of, 183
  for piscine gastroenterology, 250
  for reptile gastroenterology, 273–274, 277

Congenital malocclusion, in rabbits, 341–342

Contrast imaging studies, intestinal, for amphibian gastroenterology, 225
    for rabbit gastroenterology, 344, 351–352

Coprodeum, in psittacines, 322–323

Coronavirus(es), in ferrets, 205–206, 208
  in rabbits, 356–357

Corticosteroids, in psittacine gastroenterology, 330

Crop, of psittacines, anatomy of, 320
  disorders of, 325–329

Crop fistulas, in psittacines, 327–328

Crop impaction, in psittacines, 326–327

Crop stasis, in psittacines, 325–326

Cryptobia infections, gastrointestinal, in piscines, 257–258

Cryptococcus infections, gastrointestinal, in ferrets, 210

Cryptosporidiosis, in reptiles, 283–284

Culling, for M ornithogaster infection, 295, 331

Cultures, for amphibian gastroenterology, 226
  for ferret gastroenterology, 206, 210
    H mustelae sample collection, 194–200
  for psittacine gastroenterology, 334
  for reptile gastroenterology, 273–274, 280

Cystic granulomas, in amphibians, 230

Cytopathology, in amphibian gastroenterology, 225–226, 230–231
  in psittacine gastroenterology, 326, 331
  of M ornithogaster, 289–290, 292–293

D

DDT exposure, amphibian deformities from, 222, 226

Deformities, anatomic, in amphibian gastroenterology, 222, 226

Dental disease, in rabbits, 341–342

Diarrhea, in amphibians, 222, 232
  in ferrets, 203–206, 213
  in raptors, 310

Diet therapy, for gastrointestinal disease, in ferrets, 212

Digestion, in amphibians, adults, 218–221
    larvae, 217–218
  in ferrets, 187–189
    pancreas role, 176–177
  in piscines, 241–242, 244
  in psittacines, 320–321
  in raptors, 300–304
  in reptiles, 269–270

Digestive enzymes, in amphibians, 219–221
    in ferrets, 187, 189–191
    in humans, 174
    in piscines, 242
    in psittacines, 320–321
    in raptors, 303–304
    in reptiles, 271

DNA sequencing, in human
    gastroenterology, 175
        avian applications of, 182
        reptile applications of, 184
    of *H mustelae,* in ferrets, 191

Dysautonomia, intestinal, in rabbits, 361

Dysbiosis, in rabbits, 353–355

Dysphagia, in piscines, 257

E

Electron microscopy, for *M ornithogaster*
    isolation, 289–290

Endocrine function, of pancreas, in piscines,
    244

Endoparasites. See *Parasitic disease.*

Endoscopic retrograde
    cholangiopancreatography (ERCP),
    175

Endoscopy, for amphibian
    gastroenterology, 225
    for ferret gastroenterology, 211
    for human gastroenterology, 175–180
        avian applications of, 182
        capsule, 176–180
        ferret applications of, 184, 194
        reptile applications of, 184
        standard, 175–176
    for piscine gastroenterology, 250–251
    for psittacine gastroenterology, 332
    for rabbit gastroenterology, 346, 350
    for raptor gastroenterology, 306
    for reptile gastroenterology, 274

Endotoxic shock, in psittacines, 334

Enteric septicemia of catfish (ESC), 255

Enteritis, in amphibians, 222–223, 228
        bacterial, 231
        viral, 222, 231
    in ferrets, eosinophilic, 208, 211
        epizootic catarrhal, 208
        infectious, 204–208, 211
    in piscines, 257–258
    in psittacines, 335
    in reptiles, 281

Environment, management of, for *M
    ornithogaster* elimination, 294–295

Enzyme-linked immunoassay (ELISA), in
    ferret gastroenterology, 196
    in piscine gastroenterology, 253, 255
    in rabbit gastroenterology, 354
    in reptile gastroenterology, 273, 279,
        283

Eosinophilic gastroenteritis, in ferrets, 208,
    211

Epizootic catarrhal enteritis (ECE), in
    ferrets, 208

Epizootiology, in ferret gastroenterology,
    192
    in rabbit gastroenterology, 360

Escherichia coli, pathogenic, in ferret
    gastroenterology, 204, 207
    in rabbit gastroenterology, 355

Esophageal lacerations, in psittacines, 328

Esophageal sphincters, in amphibians, 219
    in ferrets, gastroesophageal reflux and,
        188–189

Esophageal stasis, in psittacines, 325–326

Esophagitis, in rabbits, 344–345

Esophagus, of amphibians, anatomy of, 219
    of piscines, anatomy of, 240, 246
        disorders of, 259
    of psittacines, anatomy of, 320
        disorders of, 325–329
    of raptors, anatomy of, 300
    of reptiles, anatomy of, 269

Eustachian tube, of reptiles, anatomy of,
    268–269

Euthanasia, in psittacine gastroenterology,
    330

Exhibit history, in piscine gastroenterology,
    247

Exocrine function, of pancreas, in ferrets,
    176–177
        in piscines, 244
        in raptors, 303–304
        in reptiles, 271

Exploratory surgery, for ferret
    gastroenterology, 204, 211–212
    for piscine gastroenterology,
        250–251

F

Facultative anaerobic bacteria. See
    Macrohabdus ornithogaster.

Famotidine, for *H mustelae* infections, in
    ferrets, 198, 200

Fat storage, in piscines, 245

Fatty liver syndrome, in piscines, 256–257

Fecal examination, for *M ornithogaster,*
   292–293
   in amphibian gastroenterology,
      223–224
   in ferret gastroenterology, 183–184,
      212
      for *H mustelae,* 195–196,
         204–205
   in human gastroenterology, 174
      avian applications of, 182
      ferret applications of, 183–184
   in piscine gastroenterology, 249–250,
      256
   in psittacine gastroenterology, 334
   in raptor gastroenterology, 310
   in reptile gastroenterology, 273, 283,
      286

Fecal-oral transmission, of *H mustelae,* 192

Feeding patterns, of amphibian larvae,
   217–218
   of piscines, 241
   of raptors, 299–300

Fenbendazole toxicity, in raptors, 308–309

Fermentation, microbial intestinal, in
   piscines, 244

Ferret gastroenterology, **187–202**
   as hypermotile and secretory, 187
   biliary system and, 176–177
   diagnosis of, 210–212
      biopsy for, 184, 204–205,
         207–208, 211–212
      clinical pathology in, 210–211
      endoscopy for, 211
      exploratory surgery for, 204,
         211–212
      miscellaneous testing in, 212
      radiography for, 204, 210
      ultrasonography for, 210
   diseases, **203–215**
      bacterial, 204–207
      diagnosis of, 210–212
      diarrhea etiologies, 203–206
      eosinophilic gastroenteritis, 208,
         211
      foreign body ingestion, 203–205,
         211
      gastric ulceration, 193, 204,
         211–212
      inflammatory, 194, 205–206,
         208–210, 213
      megaesophagus, 209, 211
      miscellaneous, 205, 209–210
      neoplasia, 205, 209, 213

         proliferative, 206, 211
         viral, 205–208
      H mustelae infections, 191–200
         diagnosis of, 174, 194–199
            immunostaining, 191,
               195–197
            sample collection for,
               194–200
         disease presentations,
            192–194
         epizootiology of, 192
         histopathology of, 191–193
         human gastroenterology
            applications for, 183–184,
               192–193
         transmission of, 192
         treatment regimens for,
            199–200
            adjunctive, 198, 200
            based on clinical trials, 198,
               200
            effectiveness related to swab
               source, 199–200
      intestine physiology, 175–176
      pancreas role, endocrine, 244
         exocrine, 176–177
      stomach physiology, 174–175
      treatment of, 212–214
         drugs for, 212–213
         neoplasia considerations, 213
         supportive care, 212

Fine-needle aspiration, in rabbit
   gastroenterology, 343, 352

Fish gastroenterology, **237–266**. See also
   Piscine gastroenterology.

Fistula(s), crop, in psittacines, 327–328

Fluconazole, for *M ornithogaster* infection,
   294

Food impaction, in amphibians, 222, 228

Foreign object ingestion, in amphibians,
   228
   in ferrets, 203–205, 211
   in piscines, 257
   in psittacines, 324, 327, 332–333
   in rabbits, 345, 350
   in reptiles, 275–277

Fundic movement, in amphibians, 219

Fungal granulomas, in amphibians, 230

Fungal infections, gastrointestinal, in
   amphibians, deformities from, 222,
   226, 229
      in reptiles, 281–282
      megabacteria as. See
         Macrohabdus ornithogaster.

G

Gall bladder, of ferrets, anatomy of, 176–177
of piscines, anatomy of, 244–245
of raptors, anatomy of, 304
of reptiles, anatomy of, 271

Gas exchange, in piscines, 245–246

Gastric contractions. See *Motility.*

Gastric dilatation, neuropathic, in psittacines, 329–330, 334

Gastric distention, in amphibians, 221, 228, 232

Gastric endoscopy, for amphibian gastroenterology, 225

Gastric hemorrhage, erosive, with *H mustelae* infections, in ferrets, 193

Gastric stasis, in rabbits, 346–350

Gastric swabs, for *H mustelae,* in ferrets, 195–199

Gastric ulcers, in ferrets, with *H mustelae* infections, 193
in rabbits, 345–346

Gastritis, infectious, in ferrets, 204–208, 211
H mustelae, 192–194
in piscines, 257–258
in reptiles, 281

Gastroenterology, amphibian, **217–235**. See also *Amphibian gastroenterology.*
ferret, **187–202, 203–215**. See also *Ferret gastroenterology.*
human, **173–185**. See also *Human gastroenterology.*
piscine, **237–266**. See also *Piscine gastroenterology.*
psittacine, **319–339**. See also *Psittacine gastroenterology.*
rabbit, **341–365**. See also *Rabbit gastroenterology.*
raptor, **297–317**. See also *Raptor gastroenterology.*
reptile, **267–288**. See also *Reptile gastroenterology.*

Gastroesophageal reflux, in ferrets, esophageal sphincters and, 188–189

Gastrostomy tubes, percutaneous, in rabbits, 350

Gastrotomy, for obstructions, in rabbits, 351

Genetics, of *Helicobacter* spp, in inflammatory bowel disease, 194, 208–209

Geophagy, in reptiles, 275–277

Giemsa stain, of *M ornithogaster,* 293

Gizzard. See *Ventriculus.*

Glottis, of reptiles, anatomy of, 268

Glucose metabolism, in piscines, 245

Glycogen metabolism, in piscines, 245

Gram stain, in ileus diagnosis, 183
in psittacine gastroenterology, 331, 334–335
of *M ornithogaster,* 292–293, 331

Granulomatous conditions, in amphibians, 229–230
neoplasia versus, 231

Guinea pigs, ileus in, 183

H

Hand-raising, of chicks, for *M ornithogaster* elimination, 295

Heavy metal toxicosis, in psittacines, 329, 331–332
in reptiles, 274

Helicobacter mustelae infection, in ferrets, 191–200
diagnosis of, 194–199, 207, 210
immunostaining, 191, 195–197
sample collection for, 194–200
disease presentations, 192–194
epizootiology of, 192, 203–205
human gastroenterology applications, 183–184, 192–193
microbiology of, 191
transmission of, 192
treatment regimens for, 199–200
adjunctive, 198, 200
based on clinical trials, 198, 200
effectiveness related to swab source, 199–200

Helicobacter pylori infection, in human gastroenterology, 174, 180–181
ferret applications of, 183–184, 192, 213

Helicobacter spp, hepatic disease role, 194
inflammatory bowel disease and, 194
in ferrets, 204–205, 208–209, 213

Hemangiosarcomas, hepatic, with *H mustelae* infections, in ferrets, 194

Hematopoietic tissue, of pancreas, in piscines, 245

Hemorrhagic erosions, gastric, with
H mustelae infections, in ferrets, 193

Hepatic disease, in piscines, 256–257
in raptors, 310–311

Hepatic hemangiosarcomas, with
H mustelae infections, in ferrets, 194

Hepatitis infections, in human
gastroenterology, 175, 194

Hepatobiliary system, of ferrets, anatomy
of, 176–177
disorders of, 194
of piscines, anatomy of, 245
disorders of, 249
of reptiles, anatomy of, 271

Hepatocytes, in piscines, 245

Herpesvirus(es), in raptors, 311
in reptiles, 278–280

Hexamita infections, gastrointestinal, in
piscines, 257–258

Hindgut fermenting mammals, ileus in, 183

Histamine, in gastrointestinal tract, of
ferrets, 189

Histology, in amphibian gastroenterology,
225–226, 230–231
in ferret gastroenterology, 205,
209–211
in piscine gastroenterology, 240,
242–246
of H mustelae infections, 191–193
sample collection in ferrets,
194–200

History taking, for amphibian
gastroenterology, 223
for piscine gastroenterology, 247–248
behavioral/husbandry, 247
exhibit, 247
medical, 247–248

Hormonal regulation, of gastrointestinal
motility, in ferrets, 189–190

Host species, for M ornithogaster, 290–292

Human gastroenterology, **173–185**
veterinary medicine applications of,
acid-peptic disorders, 178–180
antibiotics, 180–181
antigen studies, 174–175
autoimmune diseases, 175
biochemical profiles, 174
enzyme measurements, 174
H pylori, 174, 180–181
imaging, 175–178
endoscopy, 175–180

capsule, 176–180
standard, 175–176
magnetic resonance
imaging, 178
nuclear, 178
radiology, 177–178
immunosuppressive drugs, 181
in avians, 181–183
in ferrets, 183–184
in hindgut fermenting mammals,
183
in rabbits, 183
in reptiles, 184–185
infection diagnosis, 174–175
inflammatory bowel disorders,
181
motility therapy, 181
potential of, 173–174, 184–185

I

Ileus, in guinea pigs, 183
in psittacines, 333–334
in rabbits, 183, 346–350

Imaging, diagnostic, in amphibian
gastroenterology, 224–225
in ferret gastroenterology, 204,
210
in human gastroenterology,
veterinary applications of,
175–178
in piscine gastroenterology, 250
in rabbit gastroenterology, 344,
347–349, 351–352
in reptile gastroenterology,
273–274, 277

Immunostaining. See Stains and staining;
specific stain.

Immunosuppression, in human
gastroenterology, 181
in psittacine gastroenterology, 330,
335
in rabbit gastroenterology, 341
in raptor gastroenterology, 303

Impaction(s), cecal, in rabbits, 361
crop, in psittacines, 326–327

Inclusion body disease (IBD), in reptiles,
gastrointestinal, 279

Incubator hatching, for M ornithogaster
elimination, 295

Infection(s), gastrointestinal, in amphibians,
deformities from, 222, 226, 229
in avian species, bacterial
enteritis, 335
candidiasis, 325

Infection(s) (*continued*)
  ferret applications of,
    183–184
  M ornithogaster, 290–292,
    330–331
  mycobacteriosis, 334
  poxvirus, 323–324
  reptile applications of, 184
  in ferrets, bacterial, 204–207
    viral, 205–208
  in humans, antigen diagnosis of,
    174–175
  avian applications of, 182
  in piscines, coccidiosis, 254–255
    differential diagnosis of,
      259–263
    mycobacteriosis, 251–253
    pancreatic necrosis,
      253–254
    protozoal, 254–255,
      257–258
    septicemia, 245
  in raptors, 305–308
    candidiasis, 306
    hepatic, 310–311
    nematodes infection,
      306–307
    paramyxovirus, 308
    trichomoniasis, 305–306
  zoonotic potential of, 231, 252

Infectious pancreatic necrosis (IPN), in
  piscines, 253–254

Infestation(s). See *Parasitic disease; specific
  parasite.*

Inflammatory bowel disorders, in ferrets,
  194, 205–206, 208–210, 213
    Helicobacter role, 205–206,
      208–209
  in human gastroenterology, 181
    Helicobacter role, 194

Inflammatory mediators, *Helicobacter*
  infections and, 194

Insects, as food, cautions with reptiles, 275

Intestinal disorders. See *Gastroenterology.*

Intestinal dysautonomia, in rabbits, 361

Intestinal lymphoma, in ferrets, 209, 213

Intestinal tract, of amphibians, anatomy of,
  adults, 219–221
    larvae, 217–218
  of ferrets, 189–190
  of piscines, anatomy of, 242–243
    disorders of, 260–261
  of psittacines, anatomy of, 321–323
    disorders of, 333–335

of raptors, anatomy of, 301–303
of reptiles, anatomy of, 270–271

Intussusception, in amphibians, 229

Invertebrate toxins, cautions with reptiles,
  275

Iodine preparations, for *M ornithogaster*
  infection, 294
  for thyroid gland enlargement, in
    psittacines, 329

Ion transport, gastrointestinal, in
  psittacines, 323

Iron-deficiency anemia, in rabbits, 352

Itraconazole, for *M ornithogaster* infection,
  294

Ivermection, for intestinal parasitism, in
  amphibians, 227

J

Jaw anatomy. See *Mandibula; Maxilla.*

K

Ketoconazole, for *M ornithogaster*
  infection, 294

Koilin layer, in psittacine gastrointestinal
  tract, 321

L

Laboratory tests, in amphibian
  gastroenterology, 224
  in ferret gastroenterology, 210
  in human gastroenterology, 174
  in piscine gastroenterology, 248
  in reptile gastroenterology, 273–274

Lacerations, esophageal, in psittacines, 328

Lactobacillus spp, for *M ornithogaster*
  shedding, 294

Large intestines, of amphibians, anatomy
  of, 221
  of ferrets, 189–190
  of piscines, 243
  of psittacines, anatomy of, 322–323
    disorders of, 333–335
  of raptors, anatomy of, 301–303
  of reptiles, anatomy of, 270

Lawsonia intracellularis, in ferret
  gastroenterology, 205–207

Lead poisoning, in psittacines, 331–332
  in raptors, 309
  in reptiles, 274

Lip anatomy, of amphibian larvae, 217–218
    of piscines, 239

Lipid metabolism, in piscines, 245

Lipidosis, hepatic, in piscines, 256–257

Liver, of amphibians, anatomy of, 221
    of piscines, anatomy of, 244–245
        disorders of, 262
    of raptors, anatomy of, 304
        disorders of, 310–311
    of reptiles, anatomy of, 271

Liver disease. See *Hepatic entries.*

Luphenuron, for *M ornithogaster* infection,
    294

Lymphoma, intestinal, in ferrets, 209, 213

M

Macrohabdus ornithogaster, **289–296**
    acute disease presentations, 290–291
    antemortem detection of, 292–293
    chronic disease presentations, 291
    clinical disease manifestations of,
        290–292
    commercial poultry production and,
        291–292
    definitions for, 289–290
    historical perspectives, 289–290
    in psittacines, 330–331
    pathogenic factors, 290–291
    postmortem detection of, 293–294
    species affected by, 290–292
    treatment of, 294–295

Magnetic resonance imaging (MRI), for
    amphibian gastroenterology, 225
    for human gastroenterology, 178
        avian applications of, 183
    for reptile gastroenterology, 273–274,
        277

Malocclusion, congenital, in rabbits,
    341–342

Mandibula, of amphibians, deformity of,
    222
    of piscines, 239

Maxilla, of piscines, 239

Megabacteria. See *Macrohabdus
    ornithogaster.*

Megaesophagus, in ferrets, 209, 211

Metabolic bone disease, in amphibians, 232

Metamorphosis, of amphibian larvae, 218

Metazoan parasites, in amphibians, 224,
    227

Microbiology, of *H mustelae* infections,
    sample collection in ferrets, 194–200

Mite infestations, in raptors, 305

Motility, gastrointestinal, in amphibians,
    adults, 219
        larvae, 218
    in ferrets, 187, 190, 213
    in humans, 181
        avian applications of, 183
    in psittacines, 321–322
        disorders of, 325–326
    in rabbits, disorders of, 346–350,
        353
    in reptiles, 270–271

Motility therapy, in human
    gastroenterology, 181
        avian applications of, 183
    in rabbit gastroenterology, 348–349,
        351

Mouth. See *Oral cavity.*

Mucoid enteropathy, in rabbits, 360–361

Mucormycosis, in amphibians, 230

Mucosal anatomy, esophageal, in piscines,
    240
    gastric, in piscines, 242
    intestinal, in amphibians, 221
        in piscines, 243–244
        in psittacines, 322–323
            trauma to, 325
        in raptors, 302
        in reptiles, 267–268, 272

Mucosal lesions, in human
    gastroenterology, 175–176

Mucous glands, gastrointestinal, of ferrets,
    189–190
    of piscines, 240–241, 243–244
    of psittacines, 320
    of raptors, 299–300

Muscle, gastrointestinal, in piscines,
    241–244

Mycobacterial infections, gastrointestinal,
    in amphibians, 229–230
    in ferrets, 205–207
    in piscines, 251–253
    in psittacines, 334

N

Nasogastric tubes, in rabbit
    gastroenterology, 349–350

Necropsy(ies), in amphibian
    gastroenterology, 226
    in piscine gastroenterology, 252–253

Nematode infestations, in amphibians, 224, 227
   in piscines, 256
   in rabbits, 352–353, 357–358
   in raptors, 306–307
   in reptiles, 284–285
      antiparasitics for, 286

Neoplasia, gastrointestinal, in amphibians, 231
      in ferrets, 205, 209, 213
        with *H mustelae* infections, 194
      in psittacines, 325, 328, 333
      in rabbits, 352
      in raptors, 304–305, 310–311
      in reptiles, 277–278

Neuropathic gastric dilatation (NGD), in psittacines, 329–330, 334

Newcastle disease virus (NDV), in raptors, 308

Nitrogen loss, in raptor gastroenterology, 297–298

Normal flora, in cloaca, of raptors, 303

Nuclear imaging, in human gastroenterology, 178

Nutritional disorders, in amphibians, 231–232

Nystatin, for *M ornithogaster* infection, 294

O

Obstruction(s), intestinal, in psittacines, foreign body, 324, 327, 332–333
      ileus as, 333–334
   in rabbits, 350–352
   in reptiles, foreign body, 275–277

Omeprazole, for *H mustelae* infections, in ferrets, 198, 200

Oral cavity, of amphibians, anatomy of, adults, 218–219
      larvae, 217–218
   of piscines, anatomical position classification, 237–239
      disorders of, 259
   of rabbits, disorders of, 341–343
   of raptors, anatomy of, 299
   of reptiles, anatomy of, 267–268, 272

Oral papillomatosis, in rabbits, 342–343

Organ of Leydig, in piscines, 240

Oropharynx, of piscines, anatomy of, 237–239
   of psittacines, anatomy of, 319–320

   disorders of, 323–325
   of raptors, anatomy of, 299–300
      disorders of, 305–307

Overeating, in amphibians, 222, 228

P

Pancreas, of amphibians, anatomy of, 221
   of ferrets, exocrine function of, 176–177
   of piscines, anatomy of, 244
      disorders of, 253–254, 261
      exocrine function of, 244
      function of, 244–245
   of raptors, disorders of, 311
      exocrine function of, 303–304
   of reptiles, anatomy of, 271
      exocrine function of, 271

Papillomatosis, in psittacines, 325, 328, 333, 336
   in rabbits, anorectal, 361–362
      oral, 342–343

Paramyxoviruses (PMV), in raptors, 308

Parasitic disease, intestinal, cestode. See *Cestode infestations.*
      in amphibians, 223–224, 227, 230
      in piscines, 256
      in rabbits, 357–359
      in raptors, 307–308
        mite, 305
      in reptiles, 282–286
        ascarid, 285
      nematode. See *Nematode infestations.*
      trematode. See *Trematode infestations.*

Pepsinogen-secreting glands, in amphibians, 219–220

Periodic acid-Schiff stain (PAS), of *M ornithogaster,* 289, 293, 331

Peristalsis, gastrointestinal. See *Motility.*

Peritoneal disorders, in piscines, 263

Peritoneal washes/lavages, in piscine gastroenterology, 249–250

Pesticide exposure, in raptors, 310

pH, stomach, *H mustelae* infection and, 192
      in *M ornithogaster* treatment, 294
      in rabbits, 353, 355
      in raptors, 302
      in reptiles, 270–271

Pharyngotomy tubes, in rabbit gastroenterology, 349–350

Pharynx. See *Oropharynx.*

Pica, in reptiles, 275–277

Pillcam SM capsule endoscopy, in human gastroenterology, 176–180

Pinworm, in rabbits, 357–358

Piscine gastroenterology, **237–266**
   anatomy for, 237–247
      anus, 243
      cloaca, 243
      esophagus, 240
      intestines, 242–243
      liver, 244
      mouth, 237–239
      oral pharynx, 240
      pancreas, 244
      pyloric cecae, 242
      stomach, 241–242
      swimbladder, 245–246
      teeth, 239
   diagnostic workup, 247–251
      abdominal distention, 248–249
      blood chemistry screens, 249
      cloacal lavage, 249–250
      complete blood count, 249
      fecal analysis, 249–250
      history taking, 247–248
      imaging techniques, 250
      physical examination, 248
      water chemistry, 247
   differential diagnosis of, 258–264
      body condition in, 248–249
   diseases in, 251–264
      cestode infestations, 256
      coccidiosis, 254–255
      enteric septicemia of catfish, 255
      fatty liver syndrome, 256–257
      foreign body ingestions, 257
      infections, 257–258
      infectious pancreatic necrosis, 253–254
      mycobacteriosis, 251–253
      nematode infestations, 256
      protozoa infestations, 254–255, 257–258
   dysphagia etiologies, 257
   exocrine pancreas role, 244
   histology of, hepatobiliary, 244–245
      intestines, 243–244
      oral cavity, 240
      stomach, 242
      swimbladder, 246
   nutrition problems, 256–257
   physiology of, hepatobiliary, 245
      intestines, 244
      oral cavity, 241
      stomach, 242
      swimbladder, 246–247

quarantine challenges, 237, 253–254

Polymerase chain reaction (PCR), for *H mustelae* infections, in ferrets, 195–197
   in treatment monitoring, 199–200
   in amphibian gastroenterology, 225–226
   in ferret gastroenterology, 195–197, 205, 207–208, 210

Postmortem detection. See also *Necropsy(ies).*
   of *M ornithogaster,* 293–294

Poultry production, *M ornithogaster* impact on, 291–292

Poxvirus(es), avian, in psittacines, 323–324
   in raptors, 306

Prey capture, by amphibians, 218–219

Probiotics, in human gastroenterology, 181
   rabbits applications of, 354–355

Prokinetics, in human gastroenterology, 181
   avian applications of, 183
   in rabbit gastroenterology, 348, 351

Prolapse, cloacal, in amphibian, 223, 228–229

Proliferative bowel disease, in ferrets, 206, 211

Protein digestion, in amphibians, 220

Protein electrophoresis, for amphibian gastroenterology, 224

Protein sequencing, in human gastroenterology, 175
   avian applications of, 182
   reptile applications of, 184
   of *H mustelae,* in ferrets, 191

Proton-pump inhibitors (PPIs), in ferret gastroenterology, 192
   in human gastroenterology, 178–181

Protozoans, intestinal, in amphibians, 224, 227
   in piscines, 254–255, 257–258
   in reptiles, 282

Proventricular dilatation disease, in psittacines, 329–330

Proventriculus, in raptors, anatomy of, 300–302

Psittacine gastroenterology, **319–339**
   anatomy for, 319–323
      cloaca, 322–323
      crop, 320
      esophagus, 320
      large intestine, 322–323

Psittacine (*continued*)
    oropharynx, 319–320
    small intestine, 321–322
    stomach, 320–321
  cloacal disorders, 335–336
    papillomatosis, 336
    prolapse, 335–336
  esophageal/crop disorders, 325–329
    fistulas, 327–328
    foreign body ingestion, 327
    impaction, 326–327
    neoplasia, 328
    papillomatosis, 328
    stasis, 325–326, 329
    trauma, 327–328
  heavy metal toxicosis and, 329,
    331–332
  intestinal disorders, 333–335
    enteritis, 335
    ileus, 333–334
    mycobacteriosis, 334
  neuropathic gastric dilatation, 329–330
  oropharynx disorders, 323–325
    avian poxvirus infection, 323–324
    candidiasis, 325
    hypovitaminosis A, 324
    neoplasia, 325
    papillomatosis, 325
    trauma, 324
  proventriculus/ventriculus disorders,
    329–333
    dilatation, 329–330
    Macrorhabdus ornithogaster,
      330–331
    neoplasia, 333
    obstruction, 332–333
    papillomatosis, 333
    toxicities, 331–332
  thyroid gland enlargement and,
    328–329

Pyloric cecae, of piscines, anatomy of, 242

Pyloric movement, in amphibians, 219

Pyloric sphincters, in amphibians, 220–221

Pyloric ulcers, in rabbits, 345

Q

Quarantine, of piscines, gastroenterology
  challenges of, 237, 253–254

R

Rabbit gastroenterology, **341–365**
  esophagitis, 344–345
  human bacterial infections and, 183
  intestinal tract disorders, 353–362
    anorectal papilloma, 361–362

    bacterial enteritis, 353–356
    cecal impaction, 361
    dysautonomia, 361
    ileus, 183, 346–350
    mucoid enteropathy, 360–361
    neoplasia, 352
    parasitic enteritis, 357–359
    viral enteritis, 356–357
  oral cavity disorders, 341–343
    dental disease, 341–342
    papillomatosis, 342–343
    salivary gland necrosis, 343
    sialoadenitis, 343
  stomach disorders, 345–353
    nematodes, 352–353
    neoplasia, 352
    obstruction, 350–352
    stasis, 346–350
    ulceration, 345–346

Radiography, for amphibian
  gastroenterology, 225
  for ferret gastroenterology, 204, 210
  for human gastroenterology, 177–178
  for piscine gastroenterology, 250
  for psittacine gastroenterology,
    329–330, 332
  for rabbit gastroenterology, 344,
    347–349, 351
  for reptile gastroenterology, 273–274,
    277

Ranitidine, for *H mustelae* infections, in
  ferrets, 198, 200

Raptor gastroenterology, **297–317**
  accessory organ diseases, 310–311
    of liver, 310–311
    of pancreas, 311
  anatomy for, 297–304
    accessory organs, 303–304
    disease classification based on,
      297–298
    lower gastrointestinal system,
      300–303
    species variability, 297–299
    upper gastrointestinal system,
      299–300
  diet variations, 298
  exocrine pancreas role, 176–177
  lower gastrointestinal system diseases,
    307–310
    clinical signs of, 307
    endoparasites, 307–308
    neoplasia, 310
    paramyxovirus, 308
    stool abnormalities, 303, 310
    toxin exposure, 308–310
  species variations, 297, 312
  upper gastrointestinal system diseases,
    304–307

candidiasis, 306
nematodes infection, 306–307
neoplasia, 304–305
of beak, 304–305
oropharyngeal, 305
trichomoniasis, 305–306

Rectal swabs, for *H mustelae,* in ferrets,
195–197

Rectum, of ferrets, 190
of psittacines, 322–323

Reptile gastroenterology, **267–288**
anatomy for, 267–271
common diseases, 274–286
foreign bodies, 275–277
infectious, 278–286
bacterial, 280–281
fungal, 281–282
parasitic, 282–286
viral, 278–280
neoplasia, 277–278
toxicosis, 274–275
diagnosis of, 272–274
anamnesis for, 272
physical examination in, 272
testing tiers, 273–274
exocrine pancreas role, 271
physiology of, 267–271

Ribosomal DNA (rDNA), in
M ornithogaster, 289–290

Rotavirus(es), in ferrets, gastrointestinal,
205–207
in rabbits, gastrointestinal, 356–357
in raptors, 310

Roundworms. See *Nematode infestations.*

S

Salivary glands, of piscines, 241
of psittacines, 320
of rabbits, necrosis of, 343
of reptiles, 268

Salmonella infections, gastrointestinal, in
amphibians, 231
in ferrets, 204, 207
in rabbits, 356

Schirmer tear test, in rabbit
gastroenterology, 361

Secretory cells, gastrointestinal, of
amphibians, 219–220
of ferrets, 189–190
of piscines, 242–244
of psittacines, 320
of reptiles, 268

Septicemia, in amphibians, 222, 231

Shock, circulatory, in amphibians, 222
endotoxic, in psittacines, 334

"Short tongue syndrome," in amphibians,
232

Sialoadenitis, in rabbits, 343

Silver stain, of *M ornithogaster,* 289, 293

Small intestines, of amphibians, anatomy
of, 220–221
of ferrets, 189–190
of piscines, 243
of psittacines, anatomy of, 321–322
disorders of, 333–335
of raptors, anatomy of, 301–303
of reptiles, anatomy of, 270

Spirochetosis, in raptors, 310–311

Spironucleus infections, gastrointestinal,
in piscines, 257–258

Squamous cell carcinoma, in amphibians,
231

Stains and staining, in gastroenterology, for
M ornithogaster isolation, 289–290,
292–293, 331
of ferrets, 191–192, 207
for *H mustelae* isolation,
191, 195–197
of humans, 183
of piscines, 251–252
of psittacines, 331, 334–335
of rabbits, 354, 358
of reptiles, 273–274, 279, 283

Stomach, of amphibians, anatomy of,
219–221
disorders of, 221, 225, 228, 232
use for breeding, 220
of ferrets, anatomy of, 188–189
disorders of, 192–199, 204–208,
211
of piscines, anatomy of, 241–242
disorders of, 257–260
of psittacines, anatomy, 320–321
disorders of, 329–334
of rabbit, disorders of, 345–353
of raptors, anatomy of, 300–302
of reptiles, anatomy of, 269–270
disorders of, 281

Stomach pH, *H mustelae* infection and, 192
in *M ornithogaster* treatment, 294
in rabbits, 353, 355
in raptors, 302
in reptiles, 270–271

Stomatitis, infectious, in reptiles,
280–281

Stool tests. See *Fecal examination.*

Stress, gastrointestinal disease from, in
    ferrets, 205, 213–214

Sucralfate, for *H mustelae* infections, in
    ferrets, 198, 200

Swallow mechanism, in amphibians, 219
    in piscines, 241, 257

Swimbladder, of piscines, anatomy of,
    245–246
        disorders of, 262–263

T

Tapeworm. See *Cestode infestations.*

Teeth, in amphibians, 218
    in piscines, 239–240
    in rabbits, diseases of, 341–342
    in reptiles, 268, 272

Teleost fish, gastroenterology of. See *Piscine
    gastroenterology.*

Terbinafine, for *M ornithogaster* infection,
    294

Thermal injury. See *Burns.*

Thyroid gland, enlargement of, in
    psittacines, 328–329

Tongue, of amphibians, anatomy of,
    218–219
        disorders of, 222, 226, 232
    of piscines, 240
    of psittacines, anatomy of, 319
        disorders of, 324–325
    of raptors, anatomy of, 299
        disorders of, 307
    of reptiles, anatomy of, 268–269, 272

Toxin exposure, gastrointestinal, in
    amphibians, deformities from, 222, 226
        in psittacines, 329, 331–332
        in raptors, 308–310
        in reptiles, 274

Toxoplasmosis, in raptors, 311

Trauma, in psittacine gastroenterology, 324,
    327–328
    in raptor gastroenterology, 304–305

Trematode infestations, in amphibians, 224,
    227
    in rabbits, 357–358
    in reptiles, 284

Trichomoniasis, in raptors, 305–306

Tuberculosis, in raptors, 311

Tumor suppressor genes, *Helicobacter*
    infections and, 194, 208–209

Tumors. See *Neoplasia.*

U

Ulcers, gastric, in ferrets, 204, 211–212
        with *H mustelae* infections,
        193
    in rabbits, 345–346

Ultrasonography, for amphibian
    gastroenterology, 225
    for ferret gastroenterology, 210
    for human gastroenterology,
        175–176
        avian applications of, 182
        ferret applications of, 184
    for piscine gastroenterology, 250
    for rabbit gastroenterology, 352
    for reptile gastroenterology, 273–274,
        277

Urea breath test, for *H mustelae,* 196
    for *H pylori,* 174

Urine storage, in psittacines,
    322–323

V

Ventriculus, of psittacines, anatomy,
    320–321
        disorders of, 329–333
    of raptors, anatomy of, 300–302

Viral infections, gastrointestinal, in
    amphibians, 222, 231
    in ferrets, 205–208
    in humans, 174–175
    in piscines, 253–254
    in rabbits, 356–357
    in raptors, 306, 308, 310–311
    in reptiles, 278–280
        neoplasia associated with,
        277–278

Vitamin A disorders, in amphibians, 232
    in psittacines, 324
    in raptors, 304–305

Vitamin D disorders, in amphibians, 232

Vitamin deficiencies, in amphibians, 232

W

Warthin-Starry stain, for *H mustelae,* in
    ferrets, 191, 196

Wasting syndrome, in piscines, 249
    in psittacines, 334

Water chemistry, in piscine
    gastroenterology, 247

Water filtration, in amphibian larvae,
     217–218

Y

Yeast infections, gastrointestinal. See
     *Candidiasis; Macrohabdus
     ornithogaster.*

Z

Zinc poisoning, in psittacines,
     331–332

Zoonoses, in piscine gastroenterology,
     252
     Salmonella as,
          231

Changing Your Address?

Make sure your subscription changes too! When you notify us of your new address, you can help make our job easier by including an exact copy of your Clinics label number with your old address (see illustration below.) This number identifies you to our computer system and will speed the processing of your address change. Please be sure this label number accompanies your old address and your corrected address—you can send an old Clinics label with your number on it or just copy it exactly and send it to the address listed below.

We appreciate your help in our attempt to give you continuous coverage. Thank you.

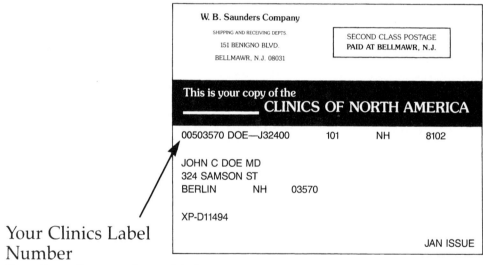

Your Clinics Label Number
Copy it exactly or send your label along with your address to:
W.B. Saunders Company, Customer Service
Orlando, FL 32887-4800
Call Toll Free 1-800-654-2452

Please allow four to six weeks for delivery of new subscriptions and for processing address changes.

8 Ways To Expand Your Practice
Step 1: Return this card.

Elsevier Clinics and Journals offer you that rare combination of up-to-date scholarly data, step-by-step techniques and authoritative insights...information you can easily apply to the situations you encounter in daily practice. You'll be better able to diagnose and treat a wider range of veterinary problems and broaden your client base.

Just indicate your choice(s) on the card below, fill out the rest of the card and drop it in the mail.

Your satisfaction is guaranteed. If you do not find that the periodical meets your expectations, write *cancel* on the invoice and return it within 30 days. You are under no further obligation.

SUBSCRIBE TODAY!
DETACH AND MAIL THIS NO-RISK CARD TODAY!

YES! Please start my subscription to the periodicals checked below with the ❑ first issue of the calendar year or ❑ current issues. If not completely satisfied with my first issue, I may write "cancel" on the invoice and return it within 30 days at no further obligation

Please Print:

Name_____

Address_____

_____

City_____ State_____

ZIP _____

Method of Payment

❑ Check (payable to **Elsevier**; add the applicable sales tax for your area)

❑ VISA ❑ MasterCard ❑ AmEx ❑ Bill me

Card number _____

Exp. date _____

Signature _____

Staple this to your purchase order to expedite delivery

*To receive in-training rate, orders must be accompanied by the name of affiliated institution, dates of residency and signature of coordinator on institution letterhead. Orders will be billed at the individual rate until proof of resident status is received.

This is not a renewal notice. Professional references may be tax-deductible.
© **Elsevier 2005.** Offer valid in U.S. only. Prices subject to change without notice. **MO 10806 DF4169**

❑ **Clinical Techniques in Equine Practice**
Volume 4 (4 issues)
Individuals $124; Institutions $209; In-training $62*

❑ **Clinical Techniques in Small Animal Practice**
Volume 10 (4 issues)
Individuals $134; Institutions $220; In-training $67*

❑ **Journal of Equine Veterinary Science**
Volume 22 (12 issues)
Individuals $171; Institutions $242; In-training $54*

❑ **Seminars in Avian and Exotic Pet Medicine**
Volume 4 (4 issues)
Individuals $116; Institutions $220; In-training $54*

❑ **Veterinary Clinics-Equine Practice**
Volume 21 (3 issues)
Individuals $145; Institutions $230

❑ **Veterinary Clinics-Exotic Animal Practice**
Volume 8 (3 issues)
Individuals $130; Institutions $215

❑ **Veterinary Clinics-Food Animal Practice**
Volume 21 (3 issues)
Individuals $115; Institutions $182

❑ **Veterinary Clinics-Small Animal Practice**
Volume 35 (6 issues)
Individuals $170; Institutions $260

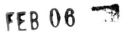

Your *Clinics* subscription just got better!

You can now access the FULL TEXT of this publication online at no additional cost! Activate your online subscription today and receive...

- Full text of all issues from 2002 to the present
- Photographs, tables, illustrations, and references
- Comprehensive search capabilities
- Links to MEDLINE and Elsevier journals

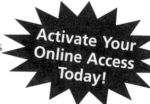

Activate Your Online Access Today!

Plus, you can also sign up for E-alerts of upcoming issues or articles that interest you, and take advantage of exclusive access to bonus features!

To activate your individual online subscription:

1. Visit our website at **www.TheClinics.com**.

2. Click on "Register" at the top of the page, and follow the instructions.

3. To activate your account, you will need your subscriber account number, which you can find on your mailing label (note: the number of digits in your subscriber account number varies from six to ten digits). See the sample below where the subscriber account number has been circled.

This is your subscriber account number

```
*******************************************3-DIGIT 001
FEB00   J0167   C7   （123456-89）  10/00   Q: 1

J.H. DOE, MD
531 MAIN ST
CENTER CITY, NY  10001-001
```

4. That's it! Your online access to the most trusted source for clinical reviews is now available.

theclinics.com

ELSEVIER